THE MYTH OF CHOLESTEROL

Dispelling the Fear and Creating Real Heart Health

Paul Dugliss, M.D.
and
Sandra Fernandez, M.S.P.H.

Library of Congress Cataloging-in-Publication Data

Dugliss, Paul, 1954-
  The myth of cholesterol : dispelling the fear and creating real heart health / Paul Dugliss and Sandra Fernandez.-- 1st American pbk. ed.
       p. ; cm.
  Includes bibliographical references and index.
  ISBN 0-9721233-7-7 (pbk. : alk. paper)
  1. Coronary heart disease--Etiology--Popular works. 2. Cholesterol--Popular works. 3. Coronary heart disease--Prevention--Popular works.
  [DNLM: 1. Cardiovascular Diseases--etiology--Popular Works. 2. Cardiovascular Diseases--prevention & control--Popular Works. 3. Hypercholesterolemia--complications--Popular Works. WG 113 D866m 2005] I. Fernandez, Sandra, 1969- II. Title.
  RC685.C6D84 2005
  616.1'23071--dc22

                                                                        2005010864

Cover Design: Ko Wicke, Proglyphics
Illustrations: Sandra Fernandez and Omari Orr

For Our Patients

CONTENTS

SECTION I: DISPELLING THE FEAR

SECTION II: CREATING HEART HEALTH

DISCLAIMER

No part of this book is intended to substitute for medical advice, diagnosis, or treatment. Every individual is unique, and therefore no book can possibly address each person's special situation. Do not make changes in your medications or lifestyle without consulting your health care provider. The information contained in this book is intended to stimulate discussion with your health care providers and not to replace their advice.

SECTION I:
DISPELLING THE FEAR

* 1 *

THE NEED TO KNOW

Cholesterol Blues

"I try to be so healthy. But, my labs results... I am so distraught...
MY CHOLESTEROL!"

"Forget about your cholesterol."

"You're a doctor. How can you say that! Isn't cholesterol the main
cause of heart disease?"

"No. That's not accurate."

"Doesn't cholesterol kill you?"

"That's a myth."

"What?!"

"It's a myth. Now that I have your attention, let's talk real heart facts."

Forget about cholesterol. These are the last words you expect to hear from a doctor. In counseling patients in our clinic, we realize that most are very reluctant to accept this message. This is understandable considering all they have previously heard and read about cholesterol. Given all the mental conditioning they have had, it is hard for them to accept that their cholesterol levels are only minimally important. However, a close examination of the scientific research on cholesterol and heart health yields some startling revelations. Focusing on cholesterol has actually detracted from promoting real heart health. How did we get to such a confused state? What are the myths about cholesterol that have become ingrained in our culture? What does an informed person need to know to take care of his or her heart?

> **Myth Defined:**
> **2a**: a popular belief or tradition that has grown up around something or someone; *especially*: one embodying the ideals and institutions of a society or segment of society <seduced by the American *myth* of individualism — Orde Coombs>
>
> **2b**: an unfounded or false notion

Case Study: Susan

Susan has just turned 40 and, as part of her New Year's resolution, she has decided to take better care of her health. In her efforts to improve herself, she has undergone a complete physical and laboratory testing. All her results were normal except for her cholesterol. She is extremely worried about this.

"There are heart problems in my family, and I don't want to get the same thing my father has. But, I don't want to have to take medication for the rest of my life. Is there anything natural that I can do? I don't eat that badly."

"What kind of heart trouble runs in the family?"

"Well, it is just my father. He has some sort of arrhythmia."

She is asked if she knows what type of arrhythmia it is, but she does not. She knows, however, that it is well-controlled with medication.

"How old was your father when this problem started?"

"He was 76."

"So your father had no heart problems until he was 76? Is that correct?"

Susan explains that her father started having high blood pressure at age 68, and then developed the arrhythmia at age 76. According to Susan, the cardiologist said that, because he was on a diuretic for his blood pressure, his potassium got out of balance, and that might have brought out the arrhythmia.

"So how high was your cholesterol?"

"It was 240. I was told normal is below 200. I can't believe it is that high. I don't eat meat. I haven't gained weight. I am just really concerned."

She carries with her the laboratory printout of her results. Her total cholesterol is 240. Her HDL (the so-called "good" cholesterol) is 102. There is silence as the numbers are reviewed.

"What? Am I in that much trouble?" she asks.

"You have absolutely nothing to worry about. This is one of the highest HDL-cholesterols I have seen in my practice. Even if you buy into the whole cholesterol theory, you have to distinguish between 'good' and 'bad' cholesterol. Good cholesterol protects against heart disease, and it makes up a major portion of your total cholesterol."

"But my cholesterol is so high…"

"Susan, it doesn't matter. Your good cholesterol is so high that it is pushing up your total number. It is not the total number that matters. Moreover, cholesterol itself plays an insignificant role in heart disease. And you have no real risk factors for heart disease."

———

In spite of attempts to reassure her, Susan continued to worry. She called back the next day to make sure that she understood. What Susan didn't realize is that she has fallen prey to a common cultural misperception. It is not that she did not understand her results. It is, rather, that her sole focus on the numbers has distracted her from the fact that cholesterol plays a minor and, at best, indirect role in heart disease. This is

> *It takes much more than cholesterol molecules flowing through your bloodstream to cause heart disease.*

the case particularly for a person like Susan who has no other risk factors for heart disease — she doesn't smoke; she is not overweight; she does not have diabetes; she does not have high blood pressure. The fact of the matter is this: Her worry and anxiety about her cholesterol is creating more damage to her heart than her cholesterol ever will. It takes a lot more than cholesterol molecules flowing through your circulatory system to cause heart disease.

———

It is for Susan and others like her that we write a book that challenges "the myth of cholesterol." It is time to dispel the myth by shedding light on the subject. People need to know. The singular focus on "my cholesterol number" is actually keeping people sick. It has created a cultural anxiety about this issue. This, in turn, has only served to spurn a boon in the pharmaceutical industry. Few others have benefited. More insidiously, though, is the fact that it has distracted people from taking the necessary steps to promote heart health. They have turned their attention away from creating overall health, in favor of focusing exclusively on one aspect of the cardiovascular system.

> *Few people know that cholesterol, in and of itself, is benign.*

We became aware of the tremendous need for education to counter prevalent cultural perceptions in our Preventive Medicine Seminars. In one of our classes we give a 10-question quiz about heart health. The questions were chosen to challenge the reader about his or her misconceptions regarding cholesterol and heart disease. Rarely would anyone get close to half of the multiple-choice questions correct (and we often have well-educated, well-read health professionals in the audience). We realized the problem was not a lack of understanding. The problem is one of mis-education. Important research is virtually unknown to the public and much of what is disseminated is distorted. Even worse, many studies have been ignored, so that it is nearly impossible to discern the evidence-based truth.

This book intends to enlighten readers about cholesterol and heart disease. Armed with factual knowledge, it may give you cause to challenge your physician. But, more importantly, it may give you pause before refilling your prescription for cholesterol medication.

This book will provide a new perspective on heart health and disease by identifying the real culprits of this phenomenon. As will be explained, except for some rare genetic forms of cholesterol dysfunction, cholesterol is benign. Focusing on "lowering your cholesterol number" only serves to create a false sense of security. Like constantly checking that the gutters

> *Cholesterol plays at most a minor role in heart disease.*

of the house are in good shape, this preoccupation has caused us to miss the real danger — the foundation of the house may be crumbling.

The current situation in the United States in terms of cardiovascular disease is a case in point. In spite of decades of promoting cholesterol medication and cholesterol-lowering diets, heart disease remains the number one killer. Certainly, something has been missed. With heart disease at epidemic proportions, people need to know how to create and maintain heart health throughout their lives.

First, and foremost, they need to know that cholesterol plays at most a minor role in heart disease. It is far from the main factor. However, this has both good and bad implications. The good news is that you, like Susan, may not need to obsess about your cholesterol levels. The bad news is this: Low cholesterol levels don't necessarily protect you against heart disease. Other factors play a *huge* role in maintaining heart health.

Second, we encourage patients not to fall prey to the notion that health can be bought in a pill, whether natural or synthetically-derived. Unfortunately, the myth of cholesterol lends itself to the notion of "Health in a Bottle" — pop a pill, lower your number ... forget about it! This easy prescription for "health" is deadly dangerous. Because the human body is incredibly complex, a pill will only influence a very limited aspect of the circulatory system and its functioning. Many medications only alter symptoms. Rarely do they actually improve the condition of the heart and its vessels, or create well-being.

Finally, we want people to be aware of the wide range of natural interventions available to them. These are inexpensive, proven means to create heart health. The affect of these interventions will be measured in terms of "quality of life" as well as laboratory scores. The second half of this book will offer you a road map to real heart health.

The myth of cholesterol is so commonplace in our culture that only a detailed examination of it will tell the full story. The next four chapters dissect some of the main misconceptions about cholesterol. In so doing, they reveal the whole story — the real truth. This may challenge what you know and believe. Understanding uncommon knowledge will allow you to discriminate fact from fiction.

Letting go of myths can be challenging. Given the high rates of heart disease, the number of cardiovascular deaths each year, and the dramatic failure of public health efforts, your need to know may save your life!

* 2 *

THE MYTH OF TOXICITY

The belief that cholesterol is bad and should be kept as low as possible.

The Search for the 'No-cholesterol Potato Chip'

Cholesterol is bad. Right? Nowhere is this as evident as in advertising. In the late 1980s, the craze toward low cholesterol foods was in full swing. A grocery store started advertising, "No-cholesterol Potato Chips — Now on Sale." What they failed to mention was that potatoes don't contain cholesterol, and potato chips don't usually have cholesterol, unless they are fried in animal fat. (Only animals can manufacture cholesterol.) Taking advantage of the cultural belief that cholesterol is bad may make for better potato chip sales, but it does not give a proper understanding of the body, the heart, or your health.

Cholesterol is a major component of the body. It is an integral component of cell walls. It forms the backbone of many important hormones required by the body. Examples include estrogen, testosterone, progesterone, and cortisol.[1] It is the precursor for bile acids, which are important for digestion, and for vitamin D.[2] It is chemically a ringed-carbon compound with a backbone that forms the basis for all steroid compounds in the body. It looks like this:

Cholesterol is a very important part of the body. How important is it? If you want to have a functioning brain, for example, it becomes very important. It is found in high concentration in brain tissue. Any attempt to limit it or to lower it too greatly can actually create major problems. In fact, this is a main reason that cholesterol treatment in children used to be considered controversial — children's brains are still developing, and there was concern that brain development might be stunted if cholesterol synthesis in the body was blocked. Note that sentence again. The body naturally *synthesizes* cholesterol. The liver accounts for approximately 50 percent of all cholesterol synthesis, the gut for 15 percent and the skin for a large portion of the remainder. It is so important that *virtually all cells with a nucleus in the body have the capability of synthesizing cholesterol.*[3]

The fact that cholesterol is manufactured by the body puts obvious limits on the amount you can reduce cholesterol numbers by limiting dietary intake. The body needs choles-

Cholesterol: Structure and Related Molecules

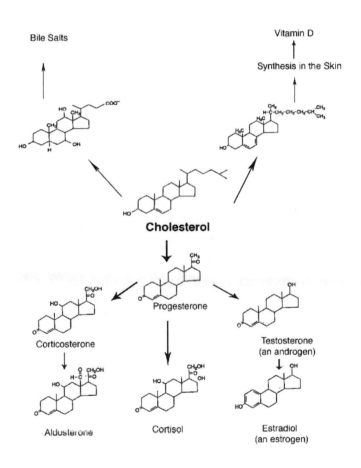

terol. It manufactures approximately 500 mg per day. It keeps cholesterol circulating in the blood. This is why, if put on a no-cholesterol diet, the blood levels of cholesterol do not go to zero. The body will manufacture what is needed for cell repair, for the creation of the hormones in the body, and other vital functions.

So important is this process that, even if you take large quantities of cholesterol in the diet, you cannot suppress its production by the body. Only the cholesterol created in the liver will be suppressed by taking in large quantities in the diet. What does this mean? Since the body manufactures about 65 percent of the cholesterol in the body, only a small portion of cholesterol production is sensitive to dietary changes. The

> *Cholesterol is so important to the body that you cannot stop its synthesis.*

body needs cholesterol and any attempt to do without it is immediately compensated. That is why study after study on cholesterol lowering via diet rarely results in reductions in blood values greater than 30 percent. In fact, the body will often compensate for low dietary intake. As less cholesterol and fats are taken in the diet, more cholesterol is manufactured by the body. The amount of cholesterol that can be reduced by diet is thus limited.

Cholesterol, in and of itself is not a "bad substance." It is needed by the body. It is part of the body and the body cannot survive without it.

The Brain Drain

Cholesterol is found in great quantities in the brain. This is not because the brain can't drain it off. It is *essential* for the proper construction of the cells that support the neurons. In fact, it has been recently demonstrated that cholesterol may play a key role in memory. This much maligned molecule is so needed for neurological function that it is actually manufactured in the brain. Cholesterol manufactured in the liver is packaged in large particles that can't cross the barrier that exists between the blood supply and the brain itself. Thus, the brain must manufacture its own cholesterol.

Duane Graveline, M.D., is an aerospace medical research scientist. He is a former astronaut and a flight surgeon. At his annual astronaut physical at the Johnson Space Center, he was prescribed Lipitor (atorvastatin), a cholesterol-lowering drug. In otherwise good health, he was prescribed this drug as a preventive measure to lower his cholesterol in the belief that this would reduce his risk of heart attack. Six weeks later, upon returning from his usual morning walk in the woods, his wife found him aimlessly walking in the driveway and yard. When she approached him, he acted confused and didn't seem to recognize her. She was able to get him to accept some cookies and milk, but he refused to enter their home. Eventually, she was able to get him to talk to one of his physician colleagues who saw him immediately and referred him to a neu-

> *Cholesterol is essential for the brain cells that support neurons.*

rologist. About six hours after the onset of his memory loss, he seemed to come to his senses. His neurologic work-up was perfectly normal, except for his amnesia. He decided to stop the drug.

The next year at his annual physical, Lipitor was once again recommended, this time at half the dose — 5 mg. Six weeks later, Graveline again had an episode of amnesia. He could not remember anything past his teenage years and did not know that he had been a family doctor, a writer, or an astronaut. Again, this episode took many hours to resolve. Graveline suspected a medication side effect from Lipitor, but neither the neurologist, nor the pharmacists he consulted would consider this a reasonable possibility. He then contacted the *People's Pharmacy*, a column that is syndicated in many newspapers across the country. He was put in touch with Beatrice Golomb, a medical researcher at UCSD College of Medicine, who had documented some cases similar to his. Meanwhile, the *People's Pharmacy* published a letter describing his reaction. Suddenly, Dr. Graveline was flooded with e-mails from patients and the families of patients who had seen amnesia, severe memory loss, confusion, and disorientation, all associated with taking drugs like Lipitor — drugs that interfere with the body's ability to synthesize cholesterol.

Graveline describes his search to understand this phenomenon in his book *Lipitor, Thief of Memory*.[4] In it he explains how scientists have discovered the role of glial cells in the brain. Neuroscientists have well-established that the brain has "plasticity." That means that as we use a certain part of the brain, the connections between nerve cells become greater in that area. If we are right-handed and start learning to play tennis with the left hand, the nerve connection in the brain responsible for movement of the left arm start to form new connections. The longer we do this, the stronger the connections. So the brain is constantly forming and reinforcing connections between neurons. These connections are called synapses.

Graveline describes how a researcher by the name of Pfrieger wanted to see if neurons could be stimulated in the laboratory to form synapses without the aid of the so-called glial cells. Glial cells are known to perform a supportive function in the brain, but their role in the formation of synapses was not clearly understood. Pfrieger attempted to grow cell cultures of neurons without glial cells. The result was that few synapses were formed. He theorized that some substance produced by the glial cells must be responsible for promoting the formation of synapses. The nature of that substance eluded scientists for years. Finally, Pfrieger's group discovered that the magic synapse-promoting substance was none other than cholesterol. Their findings were noted in the prestigious journal *Science* in November, 2001.[5]

What they discovered was that nerve cells must have external sources of cholesterol to form synaptic connections. This cannot come from the brain's blood supply or from the cholesterol synthesized in the liver, because the body packages cholesterol inside packets of lipoproteins (proteins connected to a fat particle). These packets can vary in density. The so-called "bad" cholesterol is also known as LDL or low-density lipoprotein. The "good" cholesterol is HDL or high-density lipoprotein. The catch is that even high-density lipoproteins are too large to cross the barrier between the blood supply and the brain. The brain must make its own cholesterol. And this is one of the functions of the glial cells.

For a drug to pass the blood-brain barrier, it must be lipophilic, or dissolve easily in fatty substances. Certain cholesterol-lowering drugs are small enough molecules to pass the blood-brain barrier and are lipophilic in nature. Those drugs are atorvastatin (Lipitor), simvastatin (Zocor), and lovastatin (Mevacor). The overwhelming majority of adverse drug effects affecting memory and cognition were associated with these drugs — the ones that could easily pass through the blood-brain barrier.[6]

In his book Graveline details how memory loss, depression, and cognitive dysfunction associated with cholesterol-lowering medications seem to be much more common than is reported in the medical literature. Understanding that cholesterol is not "bad," and that it plays an important function in the brain, is too often overlooked by both physicians and the general public. Graveline's book is an excellent wake-up call for us to reassess our attitudes about cholesterol.

Measure Me, Rate Me — Is Your Health the Sum of Your Numbers?

John L. brings into my office two sets of cholesterol readings. He explains that he was very concerned about his cholesterol levels being high and has been working for the last six months to decrease the amount of cholesterol in his diet.

"I am discouraged. My second reading was even worse than my first. I don't want to take drugs for the rest of my life."

He has come to my office because he is interested in alternative medicine and he is looking for a natural approach to addressing his cholesterol "problem." I ask to see his lab results. His first readings show the following:

TOTAL CHOLESTEROL   212
HDL-CHOLESTEROL   48
LDL-CHOLESTEROL   128
TRYGLYCERIDES   205

His second reading, taken six month later, shows the following:

TOTAL CHOLESTEROL   228
HDL-CHOLESTEROL   52
LDL-CHOLESTEROL   127
TRYGLCERIDES   220

From the numbers it is easy to see why John might be discouraged. His cholesterol has gone up from 212 to 228. Certainly, if we assume that cholesterol is bad, John is failing. His efforts have not paid off. Is this so? Is there any help for him?

First, even if we suppose for a moment that cholesterol itself is a problem, we have to distinguish between cholesterol that is being transported away from cells to be disposed of in the liver (HDL-cholesterol) and cholesterol transported to the cells (LDL-cholesterol). HDL-cholesterol levels are *protective* against heart disease. The higher the better. So the only real way to know anything from a cholesterol reading is to look

> *Knowing only your total cholesterol is of little benefit.*

at the ratio of total cholesterol to HDL-cholesterol — the so-called risk ratio. In May John's risk ratio was 4.4. In November it is still 4.4. This represents no significant change, even if we accept that cholesterol levels have anything to do with risk of heart disease. It does not do much good to know your total cholesterol. It is important to know the amount of HDL cholesterol that is present in relation to the total. And John's risk ratio is actually quite good. According to this measure, his risk is below average.

Second, any laboratory test has a margin of error. This means that if you take the same person and measure their blood more than once, there will be some variation, just because the measurement of small amount of a biochemical substance in a small amount of blood is not precise. Even if there is precision in the measurement, levels vary within an individual on a moment-to-moment basis. Cholesterol measurements from the same individual taken more than once will vary anywhere from 4 to 10 percent. That means that John's second total cholesterol of 228 might be actually 22.8 points lower. Likewise, his first reading might have been 21.2 points higher than the value we got. The two readings (228 and 212) are so close that we don't really know how much they have changed. But we don't care, anyway. Why? Because it is the risk ratio that is the only useful information we get from the cholesterol levels. Besides, as we will see, cholesterol has little to do with the risk of heart disease anyway.

The risk ratio has very little to offer in evaluating heart health without other information. As we will see later in the book, a bad risk ratio contributes minimally to heart disease without other factors being present. What are those factors? It just happens that most of them relate to the potential to oxidize cholesterol and create inflammation in the body, which we explain in the next chapter. That is why the emphasis on cholesterol levels alone is misleading.

This myth that cholesterol is a bad thing has had disastrous consequences. It has caused people like John to focus on avoiding cholesterol in the diet, when in fact there are many other important lifestyle changes that he could have made to improve the health of his heart and his arteries. It has also caused many people like John to be put on cholesterol lowering medication, unnecessarily — John has no other risk factors for heart disease. Medications have side effects and the widespread use of medication assures that some individuals will be adversely affected.

This is not a minor consideration. In a study published in the *Journal of the American Medical Association* in 1998, the known adverse effects of drugs were estimated to cause more than 106,000 deaths per year.[7] We erroneously assume that a medication that causes death would never get approval by the Food and Drug Administration (FDA). Think again. Baycol, a cholesterol-lowering medication, had to be pulled off the market in 2000 because it caused rhabdomyalosis (muscle destruction) and death in five individuals. And many of the currently approved drugs are known to cause problems with liver dysfunction in some individuals. More will be discussed on the problems of drugs later in the book.

> *The known adverse effects of drugs cause more than 106,000 deaths annually.*

While medications present their own unique set of problems, they have also put the emphasis on taking a pill in order to become healthy. This emphasis has shifted the focus away from the more important changes individuals can make to improve their health and has continued the illusion that health comes from pills. It has created a false rating system. People falsely believe that if their number is good, they don't need to be concerned about heart and artery health. Conversely, if the number is bad, they mistakenly believe that lowering it is all they need to do. This myth does a great disservice by oversimplifying health and catering to people's desire to rate themselves based on laboratory results.

Cholesterol isn't bad. If you do happen to have your cholesterol checked, there are some important things to know about the test before you start rating yourself:

- Illness, drugs, seasonal variation, and the position in which blood is obtained all affect the outcome
- Cholesterol values are 8% higher in the winter than summer.
- Cholesterol levels are 5% lower if the blood sample is drawn sitting versus standing.
- Levels are 10-15% different when drawn lying down versus standing.
- Levels should be drawn after fasting for 12-14 hours.
- Levels will be elevated in hypothyroidism.
- Anabolic steroids, corticosteroids, diuretics, and progestins can all elevate levels.
- The variation within an individual is normally 4-10%.
- Infection and inflammation can decrease blood sample readings of cholesterol.
- HDL-cholesterol varies within an individual by 3.6-12.4%.
- Triglycerides can vary as much as 12-40% within an individual, and the analysis of the blood itself varies from 5-10% on the same sample.[8]

Knowing that your levels can vary greatly and that other conditions can falsely elevate your readings can help you to put your cholesterol results in context. Even then, as you will see, measuring cholesterol levels is of little value. Although cholesterol an important part of the body, it is a very poor predictor of heart and artery disease.

A Slightly High-Cholesterol Diet

There is a tribe by the name of the Masai in Africa who are basically sheepherders. Traditionally, the young men live off milk, meat, and blood. They often consume a gallon of milk a day. This level of saturated fat and cholesterol intake would horrify almost any cardiologist. Yet, the incidence of heart disease is very low in the Masai. Likewise, the Inuit traditionally have consumed an extremely high-cholesterol diet, with a large portion of their calories coming from whale blubber. The Inuit, when on their traditional diet, have a low incidence of heart disease. Cholesterol and saturated fat, therefore, cannot necessarily be toxic to the human body. Even animal research supports this fact.

When animal arteries are injected with purified cholesterol, they do not develop any atherosclerosis.[9] Cholesterol is simply not a toxic substance, unless you do something to it to make it toxic. In fact, feeding huge amounts of cholesterol and fat to rabbits is necessary to create artery changes and these changes are not at all like those of atherosclerosis in humans. The artery layers become more fatty rather than calcified and thickened.

Unlike what most people have heard, pure cholesterol is a benign substance. It is part of the body and supports many of its functions.

Simply Part of the Body

Cholesterol is part of the body and a necessary part at that. Belief that it is toxic is unfounded and therefore must be re-examined. It is important to dispel the myth that cholesterol is bad. Much of this reputation has been created by the notion that cholesterol *causes* atherosclerosis and heart disease. This is another one of the common myths of modern medicine and is the subject of our next chapter.

Just the Facts

Here is a summary of the important points in this chapter:

- Cholesterol is made by almost all cells in the human body that have a nucleus, as is the case with animals in general.
- Cholesterol is needed to make sex hormones like estrogen and testosterone.
- Cholesterol is needed to make other important hormones like cortisol.
- Cholesterol is the precursor for vitamin D.

- Cholesterol is abundant in the brain.

- Cholesterol is needed by the supportive cells within the brain (glial cells) to help neurons form connections (synaptic junctions).

- Cholesterol-lowering medications that cross the blood-brain barrier sometimes cause problems in thinking and memory.

- Cholesterol readings can vary widely.

- Total cholesterol is a meaningless number without knowing the amount of HDL-cholesterol that is present.

- The body manufactures approximately 65% of the cholesterol that circulates in the blood and appears on a lab report.

- Cholesterol is not a toxic substance and does not cause artery disease, even when injected directly into the arteries of animals.

* 3 *
THE MYTH OF CAUSALITY

*The belief that cholesterol causes atherosclerosis and conse-
quently heart disease.*

How did cholesterol get such a bad reputation? Part of the
answer lies in the approach taken by modern medicine. This
began with the acceptance of Pasteur's "Germ Theory of
Disease." Through experimentation, Pasteur discerned a
cause-and-effect relationship between a particular germ and
a given disease. In so doing, he proved that the causative
agent in certain diseases was a microbe.

Since then, the scientific community's approach to "good science" has been to focus on determining a single cause for a
given disease. This approach works quite well for most infectious diseases and some genetic diseases. Malaria, for example, is caused by a parasite that is carried by mosquitoes. Both

the parasite and the mosquito were isolated. A single cause was identified. Moreover, without the parasite or the mosquito (the cause), the disease is not produced (the effect).

This reasoning begins to falter when applied to most other diseases. Causation is not so straightforward, especially in the case of modern, chronic diseases like cancer and heart disease. Moreover, it is reported that Pasteur himself re-evaluated his germ theory in later years. He is believed to have said: "It is not the germ; it is the terrain." This statement opens the door for a deeper analysis of disease causation, taking into account the significant role played by the individual's general health (the "terrain").

The Case Against Cholesterol

While searching for "the cause" of heart disease, pathologists noticed that blood vessels were clogged with plaques and debris. These plaques were areas of hardness with a mushy center; hence, the term atherosclerosis from the Greek words *atheroma* meaning "gruel" and *sklerosis* meaning "hardening." They later determined that the mushy center had a high concentration of cholesterol. Logic followed: Since the narrowing of arteries was caused by atherosclerosis, and cholesterol was at the center of these plaques, cholesterol must be the cause of the disease. The culprit had been found. This circumstantial evidence seemed enough to convict the criminal for life.

This line of reasoning is analogous to the following: A pipe in your house breaks. You look inside the pipe and see a white crusty buildup of calcium phosphate compounds. You see that the buildup is greater particularly where the pipe snapped. Did the buildup cause the pipe to break? Of course not. The more likely explanation is that there was a defect in the pipe that allowed for more calcium phosphate to collect at that point. That is all. The buildup was a symptom of the problem, not the cause.

The Lipid Hypothesis

If cholesterol, in and of itself, is not a toxic substance, how did it get such a bad reputation? Throughout the history of science and medicine, scientists have postulated other theories to explain the origin of atherosclerotic plaques in the circulatory system. Rudolph Virchow, now considered the father of modern pathology by many, thought atherosclerosis was the result of an infection, not cholesterol.

Virchow introduced light microscopy to the study of diseased tissue. He noticed the presence of immune system cells and other signs of inflammation within the atherosclerotic plaque. He deduced, therefore, that some infectious process had taken hold of the diseased area. As we will see later, Virchow's observations are highly relevant to our current understanding of what really clogs arteries.

Virchow's theories were ignored by some of his peers. In the first decade of the 1900s, a Russian scientist astutely observed that the most severe atherosclerosis occurred in members of the wealthy class.   In his book *The Homocysteine Revolution,* Kilmer McCully, M.D., describes how a Russian researcher by the name of Ignatovsky suspected that the cause of heart disease was some factor in the diet of the wealthy. Unlike their less wealthy counterparts who ate rough, unprocessed foods, the diet of the wealthy consisted of more refined foods with a large quantity of animal protein and fat. He proceeded to test his hypothesis.

Ignatovsky fed a protein-rich diet to rabbits. He soon observed plaque buildup in pathology specimens. He had succeeded in inducing atherosclerosis in the animals by only introducing dietary changes. Ignatovsky published his find-ings: A high-protein diet was the cause of atherosclerosis. His theory, however, was called into question when Ashoff, a German pathologist, discovered that fat and cholesterol were a major component of the diseased portion of the arteries in such rabbits. The focus was, once again, shifted away from the inflammation or protein theories. Cholesterol regained its place in center stage.

The primacy of the lipid theory was also the result of some failed experiments by Harry Newburgh. He surmised that cholesterol was a benign substance because it is ubiquitously present in the body. He set out to repeat Ignatovsky's rabbit experiments.

Newburgh's results unequivocally showed a relationship between high doses of protein and the formation of plaques: the higher the intake of protein, the higher the quantity of plaques. To further prove his protein theory, he set out to give the rabbits individual amino acids rather than the whole protein. Amino acids, after all, are the building blocks of protein. Unfortunately, when he did so, none of his rabbits developed significant atherosclerosis. Unable to prove that the building blocks of protein cause plaque formation, he could not logically prove the relationship between high-protein diet and artery disease. As his rabbits had not developed atherosclerosis on a diet of amino acids, he was forced to drop this line of inquiry.

> *Newburgh's results showed a direct relationship between high doses of protein and atherosclerosis.*

In retrospect, Newburgh failed through no fault of his own. The problem was that in 1922, two important amino acids had not been discovered. These two amino acids were missing from the diet he fed to the rabbits. The first was methionine and the second was homocysteine. These two amino acids were later proven crucial in the development of plaques. Unfortunately, without proof that the building blocks of protein were involved in producing artery disease, the protein theory was dismissed. Thus, the lipid hypothesis became the prevalent dogma: Lipids (fats, oils, and cholesterol) cause heart disease.

Corroborating evidence for the lipid hypothesis later came from epidemiological studies. These studies provided the following observations:

- *Some* countries where cholesterol levels are high seemed to have high rates of heart disease.

- Individuals with high cholesterol *seemed* more at-risk for heart disease than those with low cholesterol. Those with a cholesterol level of 300 mg/dL have a four- to five-fold greater risk of heart disease than those with a cholesterol level of 180 mg/dL.

- Using cholesterol-lowering drugs decreases the risk of heart attack.[1]

At first glance, the case against cholesterol appears solidly grounded. But upon further analysis, it becomes evident that circumstantial evidence is being used to convict an otherwise innocent bystander.   Let us revisit the evidence.

Pick Your Nation

Some of the circumstantial evidence was provided in a paper published by Ancel Keys in 1953. Director of the Laboratory of Physiological Hygiene at the University of Minnesota, Keys presented his opinion that public health should direct its attention to combating the increasing incidence of heart disease. He noted that four to five times as many Americans die of heart attacks as do Italians. He was convinced that this was due to the high fat intake of most Americans. To bolster his opinion, he published data on the dietary intake of seven countries. The data demonstrated a strong correlation between fat intake and heart disease.

His evaluation had a major shortcoming. Even though data from 22 different countries were available at the time, Keys omitted 15 countries from his analysis. If he had included them all, he would have found no correlation whatsoever between cholesterol levels and heart disease. Some countries, such as France, have a high intake of fat and cholesterol and a low incidence of heart disease. Some attribute this to the wine that the French drink. But, other countries that consume less wine and more fat than France had an even lower incidence of heart disease — those countries were Holland and Norway. (Sorry, it is not the wine!) Certainly, if fat and cholesterol consumption is the direct cause of heart disease, the above observations become hard to explain.

Many people with high total cholesterol have no increased risk of heart disease.

Another weakness of the lipid hypothesis is this: Many individuals with high cholesterol levels have no increased risk of heart disease. Since the lipid hypothesis was formulated, scientists have continued to find one group after another that has high cholesterol but a low risk of heart disease. These are people like Susan, in Chapter 1. Such individuals have high cholesterol, but most of the cholesterol is HDL-cholesterol.

Medical researchers recognize that the body packages choles-terol with other fatty substances in spherical structures called lipoproteins (see diagram). Some are manufactured by the body and circulated in the blood to cells that need them (LDL-cholesterol). Others seem to be coming back from the cells to the liver for processing (HDL-cholesterol). When they analyzed the difference between these lipoproteins, they found that they varied in their composition and density. Those coming from the liver to the cells are of low density. Those coming back from the cells and tissues to the liver are of high density. Hence, they noticed that those spheres with low-density lipoproteins (LDL-cholesterol) were associated with more with artery disease, and those with high-density lipoproteins (HDL-cholesterol) were associated with less dis-ease. This observation was so consistent that they revised the

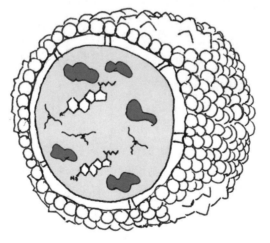

Lipoprotein Cross Section

Since oil and water do not mix, there needs to be a way to transport lipids (mainly oils) in the blood (mainly water). Lipoprotein encases the lipids so that they can be transported in the blood.

lipid theory to reflect this observation. Apparently, high levels of HDL-cholesterol actually prevent heart disease.

All of a sudden the story had to change. Now there was "good" cholesterol and "bad" cholesterol. A new campaign to educate the public and the medical profession was undertaken. This time it was to help people distinguish between the two. That campaign was not very successful. People still become tremendously worried when they receive their total cholesterol results, and the reading is above average. What they may not be aware of is that perhaps a large fraction of their total cholesterol is "good" cholesterol (HDL-cholesterol), and very little of it is "bad" cholesterol (LDL-cholesterol). As in the case of Susan in the first chapter, her total cholesterol is largely "good" cholesterol, putting her at low risk of heart disease.

An Exception to the Rule: The Italian LDL-Cholesterol

Punching an even bigger hole in the lipid hypothesis is the example of those who have high levels of "bad" cholesterol but no heart disease. How do you explain that phenomenon? A population in Italy was found to have high total cholesterol levels mainly composed of LDL-cholesterol. But, in this population, the incidence of heart disease is very low. Scientists have found that the LDL-cholesterol produced by these individuals is lighter and therefore floats even better. Researchers have noticed that it seems to actually scrape plaque off arteries rather than depositing it. Of note, this information is actually being used by a bioengineering company in Ann Arbor, Michigan, to create an intravenous solution of LDL-cholesterol that can serve as "Drano" to cleanse out diseased arteries. Scientists would be hard-pressed to defend their prejudice against "bad" cholesterol when, in fact, the "Italian" LDL-cholesterol can be used to prevent heart disease.

Look, Ma: Low Cholesterol, Bad Disease

Another way to scrutinize the lipid hypothesis is to ask if people with low cholesterol levels get atherosclerosis and heart disease. The answer is: certainly! Many people with low cholesterol levels have heart attacks. This is a major point of a book on cholesterol by Dr. Uffe Ravnskov.[2] He describes a study done by Medalie observing more than 10,000 people over a period of five years. Of the 128 heart attacks that occurred, 68 occurred in people with low or average cholesterol levels and only 60 occurred in those with a total cholesterol greater than 220 mg/dL. Twenty-nine heart attacks occurred in those with cholesterol levels less than 190 mg/dL.[3] This is just one example of many studies that show unequivocally that people with low cholesterol do get heart attacks. Certainly, this doesn't fit well with the lipid hypothesis.

We also know, for example, that people with low levels of cholesterol and high levels of homocysteine get heart disease. So important is homocysteine that it is considered an independent predictor of heart disease. This means that it correlated with appearance of disease, independent of cholesterol levels. For this reason, some physicians have started checking this when they do blood work for cholesterol.

What does homocysteine do? It damages endothelial cells and gets the whole process of atherosclerosis started. In fact, it is much more likely to be the *causative* factor of heart disease, rather than cholesterol. Homocysteine may be the *real* culprit. A major piece of evidence: It is carried in the LDL particles along with cholesterol, but not in the HDL particles. This fact may explain why LDL is minimally associated with heart disease and HDL is not.

> *The correlation between cholesterol levels and heart disease is weak at best.*

The fact that many countries have above-average cholesterol levels and low levels of heart disease flies in the face of the lipid hypothesis. Similarly, the fact that individuals with low cholesterol get heart disease certainly does not add support to the hypothesis either. Lastly, and more importantly, we have hinted at a more likely suspect, homocysteine. But, you are not yet ready to acquit cholesterol. You ask: How do we explain the fact that people with cholesterol over 300 have a four- to five-fold risk of heart disease?

All in the Family

Some cholesterol elevations are truly extraordinary. Cholesterol levels in the high 300s, 400s, and even higher occur in certain families. These families have a genetic defect. They pass on a gene to their offspring that alters the proper functioning of cholesterol regulation in the liver (at the manufacturing level). The so-called LDL-receptor in liver cells is defective. This results in cells not being able to regulate levels as the rest of us do. The individuals in families with these receptor defects do tend to have an increase in the incidence of heart attacks and heart disease. This disease is called familial hypercholesterolemia. But obviously, individuals with this genetic defect in metabolism are a special case. When such metabolic defects are in place, usually more than one aspect of physiological functioning is likely to be altered. To generalize from such individuals to the general population is a dire mistake. But, this is precisely what was done.

Individuals with familial hypercholesterolemia were not excluded from epidemiological studies. The initial observation that individuals with cholesterol levels over 300 had a greater risk of heart disease was made including data from those with a metabolic genetic defect. Coincidently, when data from these individuals are excluded, the correlation between cholesterol and heart disease certainly goes way down. Including individuals with this genetic defect will certainly skew epidemiological data in favor of the lipid hypothesis. Nonetheless, there are those who argue that the correlation between cholesterol and heart disease is weak even when such individuals *are* included in the analysis.

After a thorough review of the medical literature, Uffe Ravn-skov, a medical doctor and expert in lipid biochemistry, insists that no study has shown a correlation stronger than 0.36.[4] This is a very small correlation in statistical terms. A correlation of 1.00 is a perfect correlation, meaning that for every increase in cholesterol there is a corresponding increase in risk. Correlations less than 0.5 are considered weak by statisticians and trivial by most clinicians. In fact, the correlation is so weak that other factors such as diabetes, smoking, obesity, and hypertension become the key risks for heart disease — not cholesterol. The positive correlations seen with cholesterol are most likely explained by the inclusion of individuals with familial hypercholesterolemia.

This would be like assuming that mucous is bad and causes deadly disease based on evidence from individuals with cystic fibrosis. Those with this genetic disease produce an excess quantity of mucous plugs. As a consequence, their lungs and other organs become gravely diseased. The point is this: We would all object if medical professionals used this rationale to put large numbers of people on medication to dry up mucous. The threat of excess mucous causing major disease applies only to cystic fibrosis patients.

Drug Magic

The last support for the lipid hypothesis comes from yet another dubious association. Otherwise stated, the claim is as follows: When drugs are given to lower cholesterol, the risk of heart attack drops *immediately*. Researchers knew that lowering cholesterol levels through diet modification took almost two years to take effect. It took this long to see plaque regression and thus a reduction in the risk of heart attack. Yet, the reduction in plaque size with drugs was almost instantaneous. Could there be something else going on? Could the drugs be affecting the plaques through a mechanism other than lowering cholesterol levels? In other words, perhaps the positive response to drugs is not due to its cholesterol-lowering effect. It may be due to some other side effect (or, more properly, side benefit) of the drug. You may skip to Chapter 5 for the more plausible explanation, if you like.

The lipid hypothesis, as attractive as it may be, is built on a house of cards. Observations of countries with elevated fat intake and their rate of heart disease was incomplete, as if selected to prove the assumption, rather than to test it. Generalizing from individuals with genetic defects is fraught with problems. And drug-effects are no proof, either. They happen too quickly to be a result of lowering cholesterol. Still, the insistence on measuring cholesterol levels to determine heart health goes on.

Before we prosecute our bodies' cholesterol, it is important to get more than just circumstantial facts. What really happens with artery disease (atherosclerosis)?

Another View of the House of Cards

The cholesterol myth is hard to dispel, in spite of these facts. It is hard to convince people that cholesterol may just be an innocent bystander in the process of artery disease. After all, they have been so fervently brainwashed to believe it is the culprit. If high cholesterol levels *really* caused heart disease then there should be a direct and strong relationship between blood cholesterol levels and the amount of atherosclerotic buildup in the arteries.

One of the first attempts to demonstrate the correlation between blood cholesterol levels and the degree of atherosclerosis was undertaken by the pathologist Kurt Lande and the biochemist Warren Sperry of the Department of Forensic Medicine at New York University in 1936. They studied individuals who had died as a result of violent deaths. These were not deaths associated with heart disease.

Lande and Sperry found *no correlation* between the amount of cholesterol in the blood of these individuals and their degree of atherosclerosis.[5] Their study was done very thoroughly. It provided strong evidence to question the current cholesterol belief system. But, they were largely ignored. The only rational criticism of the study that medical scientists could muster was that cholesterol levels in the dead must not correlate with those in the living. Is this so?

An individual's cholesterol level after death is no different than before death. A study was undertaken to prove this point. K.S. Mathur and his colleagues measured the cholesterol level shortly before death and then a varying number of hours afterwards. They found that cholesterol values were nearly the same if the blood was sampled within 16 hours of death.[6] In addition, in studying 200 people who had died from an accidental death, Mathur found no connection between cholesterol values and the degree of atherosclerosis.

J.C. Paterson followed about 800 war veterans and regularly analyzed their cholesterol levels over the years. Upon death, he also did an analysis similar to Lande and Sperry's. His visual, microscopic, and chemical analysis found no correlation between blood cholesterol and atherosclerosis.[7]

On the other hand, some autopsy studies have found a correlation between cholesterol levels and atherosclerosis. But, if we scrutinize the methodology of the studies, two major issues become apparent. These two issues can create a false correlation. First, if the study includes a lot of young people, then there will appear to be a correlation between cholesterol and atherosclerosis. Young people naturally tend to have lower cholesterol levels and their bodies have also had less time to accumulate plaque. Remember, plaque accumulation takes time. In a study that involves both young people and old people, what we see is a correlation between *age* and atherosclerosis, not cholesterol. To do the study properly individuals must be in the same age group. Second, we must be careful to exclude those individuals with outrageously high cholesterol levels (350 or higher), as they most likely represent people with familial hypercholesterolemia. Genetic errors in metabolism create unique conditions that are not usually applicable to normal populations.

Let us evaluate the famous Framingham Study to see if it reveals a direct and strong relationship between blood cholesterol levels and the amount of atherosclerotic buildup in the arteries. It, too, is fraught with problems. First of all, the statistical correlation between cholesterol levels and heart disease found was 0.36.[8] This is an unusually weak correlation; one that would normally be ignored. Generally, scientists and statisticians demand a much higher correlation before concluding that a causal relationship exists.

Beyond that, some peculiarities stand out in the methodology of the study. For example, only 127 of the 914 deceased individuals were chosen for autopsy. This does not appear to be the result of random sampling. Random sampling is a requisite of good methodology. We do not known how selection was done. This alone could skew the results.

The Framingham Study concluded in their write-up that blood cholesterol was the best predictor of atherosclerosis, even greater than age, smoking status, weight, and blood pressure. However, this statement outright contradicts other Framingham data. Other results suggest that age is the strongest predictor of heart disease; and, as we will see in the next chapter, cholesterol is the weakest predictor.

Since we are all exposed to "bad" cholesterol all the time, can cholesterol really cause artery disease? The fact that these autopsy studies do not show a strong correlation makes for great suspicion. Why do some individuals with low levels of "bad" cholesterol get clogged arteries? Why do some individuals with high cholesterol have no artery disease?

Some scientists knew that cholesterol levels did not account for the whole story and kept on searching. They theorized that high-density (HDL or good cholesterol) was what protected some individuals from heart disease. Still, there were many people with high cholesterol and low "good" cholesterol who did not have heart disease. The search continued.

Scientists analyzed certain lipoproteins and found that one of these called lipoprotein(a) seemed to be particularly adept in creating atherosclerosis. Yet, the questions remained. Why didn't every patient with high levels of this ugly lipid get heart disease? And why do many people without high levels of lipoprotein(a) end up with clogged arteries? Something was missing. A deeper understanding of the process by which arteries become clogged was needed. Again, we have to ask what really happens in artery disease and whether it is possible that cholesterol is just an innocent bystander.

> *We are all exposed to 'bad' cholesterol all the time, day in and day out.*

Cholesterol: The Good, the Bad, and the Ugly

The common notion is that cholesterol is a bad thing. It is a toxic substance. Once levels get too high in the blood, cholesterol seeps into the blood vessel walls, creating clogs and plaques. It is as if somehow when levels get too high, they spill over into the vessel walls. But, we were then asked to modify our view of this menacing substance. Cholesterol could take two forms, depending on the vehicle that carried it through the body. Suddenly, there was "bad" cholesterol carried in low-density lipoproteins (LDL-cholesterol) and "good" cholesterol carried in high-density lipoprotein (HDL-cholesterol).

The reality is, however, that the blood vessel walls are constantly exposed to cholesterol. This substance is constantly circulating in the blood. Even low cholesterol levels expose the blood vessel walls to cholesterol, day in and day out. Perhaps something happens to this innocent substance? Could cholesterol be transformed into an ugly substance through no fault of its own?

Intelligent Cells: The Inner Workings of a Blood Vessel

Atherosclerosis is the disease process by which healthy blood vessels become clogged and covered with plaque. This occurs in a sequential fashion, gradually — not overnight. Blood vessels are not just tubing (see diagram). They are like a little living organism, like a body in miniature. Blood vessel cells have muscles and undergo responses to hormones, electrical signaling, and many other substances. They are under constant surveillance by the immune system. The inner wall that is exposed to the blood itself is composed of intelligent

Anatomy of an Artery

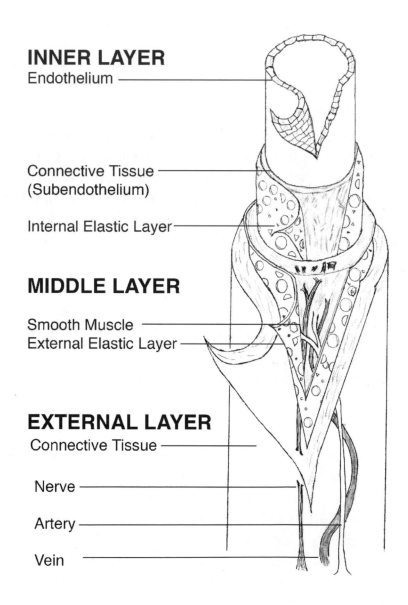

INNER LAYER
Endothelium

Connective Tissue
(Subendothelium)

Internal Elastic Layer

MIDDLE LAYER

Smooth Muscle
External Elastic Layer

EXTERNAL LAYER
Connective Tissue

Nerve

Artery

Vein

cells called *endothelial cells*. Why do we call them intelligent cells? That we will see in a moment.

Underneath the endothelial cells is an elastic layer of tissue called the *elastic lamina*. This stretchy layer allows the vessel to expand when blood is pumped through the artery. Underneath this layer exists a layer of smooth muscle. The individual muscle cells that make up this layer react to hormone-like substances to maintain and adjust blood pressure. This smooth muscle layer actually needs oxygen and a blood supply of its own. This goes to show how vital this layer is to the functioning of the entire blood vessel. Moreover, the blood in these tiny vessels is separate from the blood flowing through the center of the artery. Lastly, the smooth muscle cells are separated from the outer layer of the vessel by another stretchy layer (the *external elastic lamina*). Outside of this is a poorly defined layer of connective tissue, nerve fibers, and thin-walled nutrient vessels.

Now, what happens if the endothelial cells get damaged? It doesn't really matter how it happens. Damage could be the results from a number of sources: dramatic increase in blood pressure causing physical trauma, chemical toxins (resulting from cigarette smoke), infectious organisms, or some other toxic substance. When damage occurs, our endothelial cells send out signals alerting the immune system that help is needed to restore integrity to the wall. This is why they are called intelligent cells.

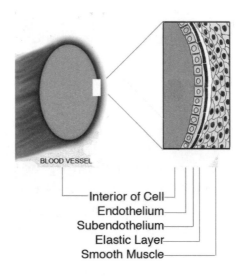

Interior of Cell
Endothelium
Subendothelium
Elastic Layer
Smooth Muscle

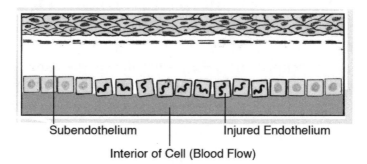

Subendothelium   Injured Endothelium

Interior of Cell (Blood Flow)

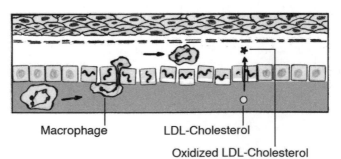

Macrophage   LDL-Cholesterol

Oxidized LDL-Cholesterol

FORMATION OF AN ATHEROSCLEROTIC PLAQUE

Initial Step: Injury to the arterial wall results in dysfunction of the cells that make up the endothelial layer.

- Wear-and-tear on the walls, free-radicals, and infectious agents can all cause injury to arterial walls. Because it is the layer in most immediate contact with blood flow, the endothelium bears the greatest impact.

- As a result of the injury, the cells that make up the endothelial layer begin to malfunction. They become unable to regulate what gets through the wall. Additionally, endothelial cells release substances that induce blood clotting and disrupt the wall's ability to expand and contract as needed.

- Surveillance cells from the immune system (monocytes) traveling in the blood can adhere to the wall and penetrate it more easily. They become lodged in the space under the endothelium. Once inside the wall, within the tissue, their name changes to "macrophages."

- "Endothelial dysfunction" is the term that describes the changes in the endothelial layer resulting from injury. Collectively, these changes are the first measurable signs of atherosclerosis.

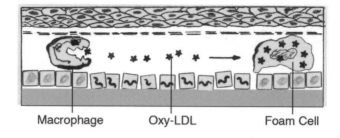

Macrophage   Oxy-LDL   Foam Cell

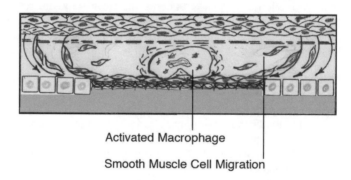

Activated Macrophage

Smooth Muscle Cell Migration

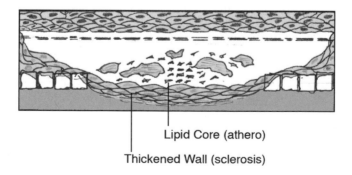

Lipid Core (athero)

Thickened Wall (sclerosis)

FORMATION OF AN ATHEROSCLEROTIC PLAQUE (cont.)

Propagating Step: When macrophages ingest oxidized LDL-cholesterol in excess, they become "foam cells" which eventually die off, releasing their contents to form a "fatty streak."

- Macrophages are big eaters. They recognize lipoproteins, attach to them, and ingest them.

- The lipoproteins reached the inside of the layer of the artery by transporting itself *through* the wall of the endothelium. In this case, however, this is a normal function of the endothelium.

- Macrophages have the ability to ingest both normal and oxidized LDL-cholesterol. But, unlike with normal LDL-cholesterol, macrophages cannot regulate their uptake of the oxidized form.

- Excessive uptake of oxidized LDL-cholesterol creates a foamy appearance to these cells when seen under the microscope; hence, the name "foam cells."

When foam cells die off, they release their contents to form a "fatty streak" along the wall of the artery. This yellowish deposit is the earliest sign of atherosclerosis visible to the naked eye upon autopsy.

Final Step: Activated macrophages release substances that eventually thicken the wall of the artery and create a protruding plaque.

- Foam cells are macrophages over-stuffed with oxidized LDL-cholesterol. When they become activated, they accumulate and release toxic substances. As a result, the artery wall is stripped of its endothelium (denudation).

- In order to repair the damage, signals are sent out to recruit platelets and stimulate the growth of smooth muscle cells. Eventually they create a hardened, thickened protrusion into the hollow center of the artery. A thin, fibrous cap is formed on top of the large lipid core, in most cases.

- The protruding plaque obstructs the passage of blood through it. But, more Importantly, the plaque can rupture and cause excessive blood loss or heart attacks and brain strokes.

The immune system responds by recruiting debris-cleaning cells to come to the site of the damage and start the cleanup and repair process. Monocytes (single nucleus immune system cells) rush to the scene. They lodge themselves between the damaged and the healthy endothelial cells. Platelets (clot forming cells) are also called into action. They cap off any open areas and keep the inside of the blood vessel's wall covered and intact.

Immune System Meets Cholesterol Molecule (Or: Ugliness Happens!)

Once the immediate threat passes, the immune cells begin a restoration process. The monocytes mature into macrophages. These immune system cells play many roles in the disease process of the artery. As they gobble up the debris, they send out messages inducing smooth muscle cells to do two things: Migrate into the damaged area and multiply.

Macrophages ingest cholesterol. Unfortunately, when the immune system meets the cholesterol molecules, bad things happen. Through a series of reactions, the immune cells manage to damage the cholesterol molecule. This molecule is then said to become "oxidized."

Oxidized molecules are criminals. Think of it this way: For the remainder of its existence, an oxidized molecule spends its time damaging those substances with which it comes in contact. No substance or cell is safe from attack.

Oxidized cholesterol induces the creation of *free radicals*. These free radicals are highly reactive molecules carrying an unpaired electron. These can damage things further by causing a cascade of reactions. But, this oxidized cholesterol is a very different beast than the normal cholesterol passing through the bloodstream. Unlike its normal self, oxidized cholesterol is implicated in at least four different damaging tasks:

- It further damages endothelial cells.
- It injures the smooth muscle tissue in the artery causing muscle cells to die.
- It promotes the transformation of macrophages into cholesterol laden giant cells (called foam cells).
- It causes the immune system to send more monocytes into the injured area.

As a result of all this destruction and attempted repairs, several changes take place. First, the passageway of the artery gets narrowed. Second, the vessel wall becomes weakened. This area then becomes vulnerable to further injury. Physical strain on this area can easily cause it to open up thereby exposing the blood supply of the smooth muscle. If this happens, the injured area bleeds. Endothelial cells are smart enough to recognize internal bleeding, so they start to recruit platelets to clot off the bleeding. Unfortunately, they are *not* smart enough to stop the process before the resulting clot completely cuts off the flow of blood through the vessel.

When the blood flow is cut off from an area of an organ, the area is prone to die. A heart attack occurs if the artery supplies the heart muscle; a stroke, if the artery supplies blood to the brain. Finally, if the growth and destruction does cause any rupture, the dead cells leave behind calcium deposits. Calcium-covered plaque lines the blood vessels thereby marking the scene of destruction.

> *In order for atherosclerosis to take place, an initial injury and an activated immune system are both required.*

This is the whole story of atherosclerosis. It requires some initial injury and an activated immune system to make it happen. In the process, an ugly character (oxidized cholesterol) is created out of an innocent bystander (cholesterol). So it is only the special form of cholesterol that is a menace to the health of the arteries.

The Cost of Free Radicals

There is a way to "scavenge" free radicals. There are substances that exist in nature that freely give electrons to oxidized molecules. In so doing, oxidized cholesterol can be transformed back into a harmless substance. That is the job of antioxidants. This has been known for many years.

The function of antioxidants was demonstrated in animals in the 1980s. Scientists took rabbits and fed them a high-fat diet. The control group received a placebo. The other group received an antioxidant called probucol. The rabbits taking probucol had a reduction in the number of regions of atherosclerosis in their blood vessels.[9] Even though the animals were genetically predisposed to high cholesterol and were fed a high-fat diet, they did not get artery disease. They were able to avoid plaque formation and calcification by taking an antioxidant.

Probucol is not a well-known drug. But, there are natural sources of antioxidants. Most of them exist in the plant kingdom. Some vitamins, such as vitamin C and vitamin E, are antioxidants as well. Could this explain why vegetarians are consistently found to have less heart disease?[10] To test this theory, many important studies were undertaken. Two of them were done in the last 10 years.

The first study showed that those taking vitamin E as antioxidant therapy had significantly lower incidence of heart attack.[11] The study further illustrated the importance of *oxidized* cholesterol in the process of heart disease. It spurned a larger, multi-center study. Unfortunately, the results were mixed.   The study showed an overall decrease in heart attacks. However, when a heart attack did occur, it was more likely to be fatal.

What can account for the mixed results? The study utilized 800 I.U. of vitamin E. At such a high dose, vitamin E can inhibit clot formation. Without clots, excessive bleeding can easily occur. Vitamin E's antioxidant effects protected against the formation of atherosclerotic plaques. However, when some diseased areas opened up and bled, the bleeding could not be stopped. The anti-clotting action of vitamin E stopped the clotting process. The result was much more bleeding and larger clots — both a prescription for more fatal heart attacks.

Most cardiologists turned their backs on antioxidants after the results of the vitamin E study. But, now there are many antioxidants that do not have an anti-clotting affect. Interestingly, some of them actually stabilize the cells responsible for clotting (platelets).

One of these antioxidant formulas has been studied extensively by Dr. Hari Sharma at The Ohio State University Medical School. It is a classical Indian formula for longevity named Maharishi Amrit Kalash (MAK). Sharma studied its free radical scavenging potential along with probucol, vitamin C, and vitamin E. The results point out the power of the synergy of herbal substances. MAK was 1,000 times as powerful in scavenging free radicals as was vitamin C or E.[12]

This would seem to make an ideal therapy for those prone to heart disease. Some cardiologists thought so and decided to give it to patients who already had heart disease. When these patients began the study, their blood vessels were severely clogged. They could not get enough oxygen to the heart muscle. Consequently, they frequently experienced episodes of angina (a squeezing sensation in their chest). After taking MAK for six months, the number of episodes of angina were more than cut in half, going from an average of 8.87 episodes per month to 3.03. Furthermore, the ability to sustain exercise improved in a third of the patient taking MAK.[13]

Even more importantly, nature has provided us with great sources of antioxidants in the fruits and vegetables we consume. The answer does not have to be in a pill or a supplement. By selecting the right diet we can get the antioxidants needed to protect against heart disease.

Unusual Suspects

Cholesterol is not a bad substance, unless it gets oxidized. It is usually just an innocent bystander caught in the heat of inflammation. Arteries do not get diseased unless they get injured and the immune system becomes involved. When the immune system gets activated, tissue damage occurs as a result of an inflammatory reaction. This is why people with high cholesterol and low inflammation have healthy arteries. On the other hand, someone with low cholesterol can get severe heart disease if, for example, they smoke and have poor diets. Smoking triggers the inflammatory process. Poor diets are generally full of free radicals and few antioxidants.

Most cholesterol in the body is not oxidized. Most injury that gets artery disease started does not involve cholesterol. But, cholesterol is not off the hook until we can point the finger at another subject. Let us take a look at some unusual suspects. Who are the truly injurious characters in this story?

1) Homocysteine

Homocysteine is an amino acid. Protein is made up of amino acids. The body is unable to synthesize the eight essential amino acids. Therefore, these must be consumed. However, the body can synthesize nonessential amino acids. It can also convert some amino acids to others. For example, methionine can be converted to cysteine. Homocysteine is created as an intermediate product in the conversion process. These amino acids are unique. Unlike most other amino acids, they contain sulfur.

This may be a lot more biochemistry than you ever wanted to know. But, this is an important process to learn about because homocysteine is toxic to arteries. It is a potent creator of atherosclerosis. This is why children with a genetic defect in the conversion process die with severe atherosclerosis before they reach their teen years. Chapter 7 will explain this issue in greater detail.

2) Stress

Stress is a mess. It creates havoc in our body. By inducing the manufacturing of certain biochemicals, it creates free radicals and indirectly causes atherosclerosis. As we will see in Chapter 6, it may be *the* greatest contributor to heart disease.

3) Hypertension

High blood pressure creates tremendous "wear and tear" on arteries particularly at branch points. The force created by the blood flow can cause small tears in the innermost lining of the arteries. Mending and repairing is undertaken by the endothelial cells and the immune system. Atherosclerotic plaques are formed in the process. Furthermore, constant "wear and tear" over time can create dysfunction in the endothelial cells themselves. Blood vessels cease functioning properly. They are unable to dilate and contract in response to signals. By causing sites of injury, hypertension is a major contributor to atherosclerosis. Chapter 10 explores this crucial point and posits that much of the hypertension we have today can be reversed with changes in diet and exercise.

4) Metabolic Syndrome

Since both endothelial injury and inflammation are required to create blood vessel disease, how important is the inflammatory process? Very important. A case in point is a recent report of a study called the WISE study (Women's Ischemic Syndrome Evaluation), which was published in a respected medical journal. In this study, researchers looked at obese women with and without the *metabolic syndrome*. Women with this syndrome have a pre-diabetic condition marked by resistance to insulin. The results of the study were conclusive. Obese women *without* the metabolic syndrome had no increased risk of death, heart attack, stroke, or congestive heart failure. Those *with* the metabolic syndrome had a *twofold increase* in their risk over the three years studied.[14] Here is the key point: This condition is associated with a known measure of inflammation in the body. High insulin in your body can induce an inflammatory response.

Moreover, insulin is known to stimulate the process of atherosclerosis. How does insulin do this? It stimulates growth factors within the vessel walls. That is one of the reasons even well-controlled diabetes (those with near-normal blood sugars) remain at-risk for heart disease and stroke. This point will be addressed in more detail in Chapter 7.

5) Smoking

Smoking is one of the most potent generators of free radicals. It creates numerous toxic chemicals that are damaging to arteries. It is a well-known contributor to heart disease. The problem is that nicotine is one of the most addicting substances in the world. Smoking cessation is a problem perhaps best handled by addressing stress. Meditation has a great potential to help with this issue as will be discussed in Chapter 6.

The Story of C-Reactive Protein

Initial injury is necessary to start artery disease. But, the immune system must get activated in order for the disease to take hold. How do we know when the immune system is involved?

Inflammation results as the immune system responds to injury. Sometimes the response can be overactive and become the source of artery disease itself. The latest effort in cardiology research is attempting to identify markers of inflammation that can be measured in the blood. C-reactive protein (CRP) has been one marker chosen for this role. In part, this is because it is one of the markers used to track other inflammatory diseases like rheumatoid arthritis.

When researchers began to notice the association of inflammation with heart disease, they decided to reinvestigate individuals who died of heart disease. This study was only possible because blood can be frozen and stored for years. Was there some clue in their blood that could have foretold that they would have problems with clogged arteries?

People with high cholesterol and low inflammation can have healthy arteries.

The scientists were able to go back and examine the blood of doctors/participants in the long-term Physicians Health Study and who had had fatal heart attacks. They thawed the blood and found a significant correlation with elevated CRP values in some individuals. A plethora of studies now confirm that when the immune system creates inflammation, the risk of heart attack is much higher.

Reality check: In individuals with high levels of CRP, the risk of heart disease is great *regardless of the cholesterol level.*

Medical practitioners have known for decades the injurious nature of inflammation on blood vessels. The impact is obvious in severe inflammatory diseases such as lupus and temporal arteritis. What has not been appreciated until recently is that low levels of inflammation can occur in blood vessels, even in the absence of systemic disease.

> *In individuals with high CRP levels, the risk of heart disease is greater regardless of cholesterol levels.*

Recall that Virchow, the "Father of Pathology," in the 1800s thought that atherosclerosis was the result of infection. He observed all the signs of inflammation under his microscope. Now we know that diabetes and pre-diabetes (or metabolic syndrome) essentially creates an inflammatory state in the body. Understanding the whole picture helps to place the topic of cholesterol in a new light.

The Real Culprits

Cholesterol, then, is not the *cause* of atherosclerosis or heart disease. Remember, cholesterol is not bad — it is a necessary part of the body. Not until it gets damaged does it become a potential source of heart disease.

Saying that cholesterol causes heart disease is like saying that blood sugar causes diabetes. It doesn't. The metabolic derangements that prevent blood sugar from being utilized by cells is what causes diabetes. That is why insulin is the cure. Likewise, artery disease is the result of a complex process, not simply cholesterol in the bloodstream.

Cholesterol is always in the bloodstream, even in people with no atherosclerosis. Then, what is the real cause of atherosclerosis? Endothelial injury and inflammation are the real culprits. For the most part, cholesterol is a passive player, a bystander at the scene of the crime. Understanding the process and the real causes of artery disease, allows us to comprehend why the results of cholesterol-lowering studies have been so confusing.

Most people are not aware that many studies have shown no benefit to lowering cholesterol. People have the opposite concept, in part, because of aggressive marketing by pharmaceutical companies and other "public education" efforts. Moreover, many of the studies showing some benefit to cholesterol lowering now clearly have other explanations.

Summary

Of all the things that can cause injury and inflammation, cholesterol seems to be at the bottom of the list. When it is involved, most of the time, it plays a secondary role. It gets recruited and transformed into a nasty character when oxidized by the cells of the immune system. But, it is something else that gets this process going. And, the secondary destructive role of oxidized cholesterol is played out *regardless* of blood cholesterol levels. This may help to explain why many people with low cholesterol levels get atherosclerosis in spite of their "good" lab results.

If you have your cholesterol levels checked, the results must be evaluated in light of other risks for heart disease. Otherwise, it is like checking the temperature gauge on your car to see how efficient your engine is running. Unless it is off the scale, it is a wasted measurement and does not tell you much. To continue the analogy, realize that just lowering the engine temperature a few degrees will have almost no impact on the life of the engine, your gas mileage, or your driving enjoyment. What do cholesterol measures mean in terms of your risk? What other risk factors are important?

* 4 *

THE MYTH OF RISK

The belief that high cholesterol puts a person at significant risk of heart disease.

Assessing Risk:

A 55-year-old male is prescribed medication to lower his cholesterol level. His cholesterol level drops from 240 to 180. By how much has this drop in cholesterol decreased his risk of a heart attack in the next 10 years? Assume he has no other risk factors for heart disease, and that his risk ratio is proportionately improved in the process.

    A. 60%

    B. 30%

    C. 20%

    D. 2%

Lowering cholesterol by 60 points can be an arduous task — one that can require multiple drugs and lots of effort. This example illustrates an important point. The answer is below.

Framing the Framingham Story

The population of the small town of Framingham, Massachusetts, has been involved in an ongoing investigation into the risk factors that contribute to heart disease.[1] Data from this population have been the foundation for many studies that have quantified the importance of various risk factors. Based on data generated from these studies, people are able to assess their risk of having a heart attack in the next five or 10 years. This information can be obtained from the table below. The American Heart Association also publishes this data, and many schemes have been developed for the purpose of assessing risk utilizing the Framingham data.

> *For many people, lowering cholesterol by 60 points only lowers the absolute risk of heart attack by 2 percent.*

Based on the information found in this table, we are astounded to realize that lowering the cholesterol level by 60 points only lowers the absolute risk of a heart attack by *2 percent*. After worrying for years about the importance of cholesterol readings, many are

AGE	POINTS			DIABETES	POINTS
30-34	-1				
35-39	0			No	0
40-44	1			Yes	2
45-49	2				
50-54	3			**SMOKER**	
55-59	4				
60-64	5			No	0
65-69	6			Yes	2
70-74	7				

LDL-Cho-lesterol	POINTS			HDL-Cho-lesterol	POINTS
<100	-3			<35	2
100-129	0			35-44	1
130-159	0			45-49	0
160-190	1			50-54	0
>190	2			>60	-1

Systolic Blood Pressure	Diastolic <80mm	Diastolic 80-84	Diastolic 85-89	Diastolic 90-99	Diastolic >100
<120	0	0	1	2	3
120-129	0	0	1	2	3
130-139	1	1	1	2	3
140-159	2	2	2	2	3
>160	3	3	3	3	3

TOTAL POINTS	10-Year CHD RISK, Percent	TOTAL POINTS	10-Year CHD RISK, Percent
<-3	1	6	11
-2	2	7	14
-1	2	8	18
0	3	9	22
1	4	10	27
2	4	11	33
3	6	12	40
4	7	13	47
5	9	>=14	>=56

To Calculate Risk Estimate: Add the points for age, presence of diabetes, smoking status, LDL-cholesterol, HDL-cholesterol, and blood pressure. Find the total point score on the bottom table to determine the 10-year risk of Coronary Heart Disease (CHD).*

*Use to calculate the risk of developing clinical coronary heart disease in men who do not have known CHD. (For additional information, see: Wilson PW, D'Aostion R, Levy D, et al, *Circulation* 1998; 97:1837.)

Table 1: Framingham Risk Score for Men

AGE	POINTS		DIABETES	POINTS
30-34	-9			
35-39	-4		No	0
40-44	0		Yes	4
45-49	3			
50-54	6		**SMOKER**	
55-59	7			
60-64	8		No	0
65-69	8		Yes	2
70-74	8			

LDL-Cho-lesterol	POINTS		HDL-Cho-lesterol	POINTS
<100	-2		<35	5
100-129	0		35-44	2
130-159	0		45-49	1
160-190	2		50-54	0
>190	2		>60	-2

Systolic Blood Pressure	Diastolic <80mm	Diastolic 80-84	Diastolic 85-89	Diastolic 90-99	Diastolic >100
<120	-3	0	0	2	3
120-129	0	0	0	2	3
130-139	0	0	0	2	3
140-159	2	2	2	2	3
>160	3	3	3	3	3

TOTAL POINTS	10-Year CHD RISK, Percent	TOTAL POINTS	10-Year CHD RISK, Percent
<-2	1	8	8
-1	2	9	9
0	2	10	11
1	3	11	13
2	3	12	15
3	3	13	17
4	4	14	20
5	5	15	24
6	6	16	27
7	7	>=17	>=32

To Calculate Risk Estimate: Add the points for age, presence of diabetes, smoking status, LDL-cholesterol, HDL-cholesterol, and blood pressure. Find the total point score on the bottom table to determine the 10-year risk of Coronary Heart Disease (CHD).*

*Use to calculate the risk of developing clinical coronary heart disease in women who do not have known CHD. (For additional information, see: Wilson PW, D'Aostion R, Levy D, et al, *Circulation* 1998; 97:1837.)

Table 2: Framingham Risk Score for Women

shocked to find that, for most people, whopping changes in cholesterol make little impact.

It is important to understand that men have higher risk than women. Therefore, in our example, if the subject had been a 55-year-old female, the absolute risk reduction would have been only *1 percent*. If our subject was a woman with an HDL-cholesterol of 68 and the same total cholesterol of 240, lowering her cholesterol to 180 would make *no impact*. The risk of having a heart attack in five or even 10 years would be 1 percent either way.

How can it be that cholesterol levels have so little impact on the risk on heart disease? Don't advertisements say that the latest cholesterol drug lowers the chance of a heart attack by 25 percent or even 50 percent? To understand this discrepancy, we need to discuss some of the terminology that is used in statistics.

Misleading Statistics

Some have described statistics as tools to manipulate the truth. That is not always the case. Often a little knowledge can go a long way in avoiding misinformation. Below is a little background on how the experts talk about risk.

Relative Risk and Absolute Risk Defined

Relative Risk: The risk of having a condition, based on comparing the number of people with that condition in each of two groups (usually a treatment group and a control group). This number is independent of the total number of people observed in the study.

Absolute Risk: The risk of having a condition based on comparing the number of people with that condition to the total number of people observed.

Relative Risk vs. Absolute Risk

Take, for example, 1,000 people from Framingham and observe them for five years. During that time 20 of them have heart attacks. The *absolute risk* of having a heart attack based on these numbers is going to be 2 percent (i.e., 20 divided by 1,000). But, most research studies do not report the absolute risk. The huge risk reductions you hear advertised on television that also serve as the rationale used by cardiologists to justify prescribing drugs are based on data using a statistical term called *relative risk*.

Here is the trick. Researchers don't compare the number of people with heart attack to the total number without heart attack (or to the number of people observed). They compare the number of heart attacks in those taking the drug to the number of heart attacks in those without the drug. Here is an example of what is done. Suppose a pharmaceutical company wants to evaluate a new drug. The drug lowers cholesterol levels and is, therefore, believed to lower the risk of heart attack. The drug is given to an experimental group composed of 1,000 people who are matched to a control group of similar age and health problems. At the end of five years, they notice that only 10 people taking the drug have had heart attacks as compared to 20 people who did not take the drugs. They declare success and state that the drugs reduced the risk of heart attack by 50 percent.

How can they say that when the rate of heart attack has gone from 2 percent to only 1 percent? This is not a 50 percent improvement in risk. It is only a 1 percent improvement in risk. How to make sense of this mess?

The researchers are not lying. They are simply viewing the results from a different perspective. They are using a different measure: *relative risk*. This measure focuses only on heart attack cases — 10 in the experimental group and 20 in the control group — and compares the two. Since 10 represents half of 20, there appears to be a whopping 50 percent reduction as a

> *The belief that cholesterol is the major risk for heart attack is simply wrong.*

result of taking the drug. Relative risk does not take into account the total number of participants in the study. Consequently, it ignores the fact that the overall risk of heart attacks might be very small for the population as a whole.

Unfortunately, most medical research reports results in terms of relative risk. To compensate for the admitted bias this creates, some studies will also report another important value:

NNT or *Number Needed to Treat.* This tells us how many people require treatment in order to help just one of them.

In our example above, we would have to treat 100 people in order to prevent one heart attack (1,000 divided by 10). That may be all well and good, if there is no downside to taking medication. Unfortunately, most drugs have side effects and are financially costly. For example, if the drug being tested creates liver problems in 2 percent of people who take it. For some of them, this could mean permanent liver damage (perhaps half of the 2 percent). Then, for every heart attack prevented by the new drug, a new case of liver disease emerges. Not a very good situation at all. Not all heart attacks are fatal. But, liver damage can create a marked decrease in the quality of life, and it can also be fatal.

Are we really better off giving the drug if it causes as many problems as it cures? This is the key point: Risk has to be interpreted *in context.*

The NNT value is important from another perspective. If the NNT for a drug is 100, then only 1 person out of 100 will be helped by the drug. In other words, 99 people will take the drug for no reason whatsoever. Ninety-nine of the 100 people would be taking the medication just on the chance that they might be the one person who could benefit from it. These are not good odds for any gambler. Do you want to take a drug "just in case"?

All Those with Significant Risk Factors Raise Your Hand

The role that hypertension, diabetes, and smoking play in creating heart disease far outweigh the impact of elevated cholesterol. In fact, as we will see, only about a third of the people with heart attacks have elevated cholesterol levels.

This may be bad news for those of us who have been complacent about our heart health because of our low cholesterol levels. Now we have to realize that given the right circumstances, we too can have a heart attack. Many studies now point out the relatively small contribution that cholesterol and fats play in the creation of heart disease. Most people with heart attacks do not have elevated cholesterol. Those who have heart attacks also have diabetes or some other major risk factor for atherosclerosis. Here is the key point: *Unless you have other risks factors for heart disease, cholesterol is not worth much concern.*

In summary, the belief that cholesterol is *the* major risk for heart attack is wrong. Cholesterol plays a minor role. The majority of people with heart attacks have other risk factors, not just elevated cholesterol. What this means is that a lot of people are being treated to prevent problems in just a few. Most people on cholesterol medication will receive no benefit from them. They were not likely to have a heart attack anyway.

Many preventive medicine experts recommend that those without risk factors check cholesterol only once every five years. This news is shocking to hear. On the other hand, for those with multiple risk factors, checking cholesterol levels adds more information to the overall picture. When that is the case, then it begs the question whether interventions should be focused on primarily lowering cholesterol or on addressing the other risks factors first.

The Most Valuable Players

Let's look at how the other risk factors enter the equation. Already mentioned are hypertension and diabetes. Of course, age is also a major player. While we are constantly bombarded with the message that "heart disease is the nation's number one killer," we don't usually evaluate this in proper context. Two-thirds of people dying from heart disease in the year 2000 were 75 or older. In fact, 90 percent were older than 65. Only 7 percent were younger than 55.[2] As we age, death becomes more likely, and certainly we are at greater risk for any number of problems.

> *Of all the risk factors discussed, cholesterol is the least important.*

With most fatal heart disease occurring in the elderly, should younger people be concerned about cholesterol? These numbers suggest that aging, rather than cholesterol, is a more important factor. Does data from the Framingham Study support this notion?

Indeed. For every two years a male ages after the age of 52, his five-year risk increases by the same amount as if his cholesterol had gone up by *20* points, say from 200 to 220. Age plays such an important role in risk that increasing your age from 50 to 65 is the equivalent of taking your cholesterol from 200 and increasing it to 330. Risk due to cholesterol levels is minor compared to aging. But then, aging can't be stopped (or, can it? See chapter 6 ...). What risk factors are truly manageable?

Let us consider the impact of hypertension. Reducing your blood pressure from 161 to a normal of 120 does as much to reduce your risk of heart attack as dropping your total cholesterol from 315 to 199. Why? High blood pressure damages endothelial cells by the overwhelming forces it creates on the vessel lining. Recall that the initial step in artery disease is damage to endothelial cells, the cells that form the inner lining of blood vessels. The immune system then becomes activated. The end result is the creation of an inflammatory state.

What about diabetes? High blood-sugar levels and excess insulin in the body is associated with high C-reactive protein levels, a measure of inflammation. Hence, one would expect this to contribute to heart disease. It does so dramatically. It is so significant that the impact of having diabetes is equivalent to elevating a woman's cholesterol level from 199 to 315. Cholesterol is a minor risk factor compared to diabetes. The good news is that the majority of diabetes in the United States is preventable. Most diabetes is related to excess weight and obesity. With weight normalization, diabetes can be prevented or cured. What are some other preventable risk factors?

Preventable Factors

Smoking is a major risk factor. Smoking creates free radicals that damage the endothelial cells in arteries. It also exposes the body to many harmful chemicals. The way it damages blood vessels fits right in with our theory of how artery disease occurs. Regardless of the level of cholesterol, if you smoke, your arteries are at risk of being damaged. Again, cholesterol is not the villain. Other inflammatory factors are the source of injury.

To further illustrate the point, let us use the example of a 70-year-old diabetic male with hypertension who smokes and has an LDL-cholesterol of 200. Reducing his cholesterol by 60 points can have an impact — as much as 9 percent risk reduction over the next 10 years. However, this impact will not be as great as if the following is done:

1) The blood pressure is brought under control;
2) Smoking is stopped; or
3) The diabetes is cured by reducing weight and exercising regularly.

By taking these steps, his risk is reduced by *34 percent,* even if his cholesterol remains unchanged. Compared with a 9 percent reduction by lowering cholesterol, this 34 percent reduction is huge. And all of these steps can be accomplished without taking drugs. Moreover, please be aware that cholesterol is the least important of all the risk factors. This statement is worth repeating: *Of all the factors we have discussed, cholesterol is the least important.*

Unless you have cholesterol levels over 300 and are in that rare group that has a genetic cholesterol problem, cholesterol plays a minor role in your risk of heart disease. In fact, cholesterol itself may eventually be dismissed as a risk factor by medical community.

In the ER

What percentage of patients who arrive to the emergency room with a heart attack have no risk factors for heart disease (i.e., do not have elevated cholesterol, hypertension, diabetes, and do not smoke)? It used to be thought that it was greater than 50 percent. In 2003, some researchers took exception to this commonly taught notion and decided to prove that it was erroneous. Their study was first published in the journal *Circulation* and commanded so much attention that it was later published in *The Journal of the American Medical Association (JAMA).*[3] They decided to analyze several large studies that had been undertaken in a prospective manner — that is, studies that had followed patients for 21 to 30 years to track the incidence of fatal and nonfatal heart attack.

These researchers looked at three sets of data. One set came from the Chicago Heart Association Detection Project in Industry (CHA), which followed a population of 35,642 men and women age 18 to 59. Another set came from the Multiple Risk Factor Intervention Trial (MRFIT), which followed 347,978 men age 35 to 57. The last and smaller sample came from the Framingham Heart Study (FS), which included 3,295 men and women age 34 to 59.

As they had set out to do, they concluded that "antecedent major CHD (coronary heart disease) risk factor exposures were very common among those who developed CHD ... [therefore] results challenge claims that CHD events commonly occur in persons without exposure to at least 1 major CHD risk factor."[4] In fact, exposure to at least one clinically elevated major risk factor ranged from 87 percent to 100 percent. However, on scrutinizing the study more carefully, problems with their conclusions become evident.

First of all, there was no available information from the CHA study or the MRFIT study about nonfatal heart attacks. This is not a minor point, since nonfatal heart attacks are more common than fatal ones. Missing more than half of all the heart attack data certainly could skew the results.

Second, they initially defined total cholesterol over 240 as a "major risk factor," but later changed their definition. Why? Based on this definition, cholesterol elevations in the MRFIT study occurred in only 35.8 percent of the men 18 to 39 with heart attacks and in only 36.5 percent of the men 40 to 59. The data from the other large study, the CHA study, was even more disappointing. Only 27.1 percent of those who died from heart attack had elevated cholesterol in the 18-39 age range, and only 30.3 percent in the 40-59 age range.

In order to make the data seem more impressive, they changed the cholesterol cutoff point. Cholesterol over 200 was determined to be a "clinically elevated major risk factor." Unfortunately, this attempt to present a more convincing picture fails to deceive us.

Since the average cholesterol level in the United States is 203, almost 50 percent of the population would be considered to have a "clinically elevated risk factor."[5] Therefore, just by chance, 50 percent of those with heart attack should have this elevated cholesterol level. This is like defining excessive height as being over 5 feet 9 inches (i.e., the height of the average American male). If we look at the number of males with excessive height who have a heart attack, lo and behold we find that more than 50 percent have this "risk factor." Obviously, being taller does not put you at a greater risk of heart attack — it is just the way the cutoff was defined. When you define the cutoff level for a risk factor in a way that includes more than half of the population, it is nearly impossible to make good conclusions about the data.

This study also presented a table of the percent of men and women with two "higher-than-favorable risk factor elevations." But, there was no analysis of the percentage of people with two of the more stringently defined major risk factors, such as hypertension, smoking, and diabetes.

Data on the cholesterol contribution to heart attacks was so disappointing that even the authors had to comment on it. They stated the following: *"Although blood lipid levels are important major CHD risk factors, a 1-sided focus on cholesterol as the major CHD risk factor cannot be justified."* They also were forced to comment on the large numbers of people who had significant cholesterol elevations but did not develop heart disease. They explained: "This study also suggested that, in these large U.S. cohorts, exposure to 1 or more of the major CHD risk factors is also highly prevalent among individuals who *did not* develop clinical CHD during the lengthy periods of follow-up."[6]

> *When the cutoff level for a risk factor is defined in a way that includes more than half of the population, good conclusions are often difficult to make.*

How weak a risk factor was cholesterol? In the CHA study, women age 18-39 had cholesterol elevation only 16 percent of the time. The highest contribution attributed to cholesterol was found in the Framingham Study. Elevated cholesterol was present 62.7 percent of the time in women aged 40-59 who had a heart attack. However, there are two issues with the Framingham Study that call this data into question. First, the Framingham Study had so many fewer participants in comparison to the other studies. Second, the estimates from the study were so much higher. For example, in the CHA study, women 40-59 had cholesterol elevation as a risk factor only

38.9 percent of the time. Think of this in terms of cholesterol levels and cutoff levels. This is not much higher than would be expected in the population. For example, in men, 25 to 30 percent will have elevations of cholesterol above 240 in the age range 40-59.[7] This means that we should expect that, even if cholesterol plays no role in creating heart attacks, 25-30 percent of individuals with heart attack should have elevated levels. If cholesterol were to play a major role, then cholesterol elevation should be seen in a very high percentage of those with heart attack. In the two larger studies, the percentages of men with elevated cholesterol was only 30.3 (CHA) and 36.5 (MRFIT) percent. This is very close to what one would expect if cholesterol played absolutely no role at all.

> *If cholesterol plays a major role in heart disease, then high cholesterol should be present in most of those with heart attack.*

What were the most important risk factors? Smoking and hypertension. Smoking was a factor in women aged 18-39 80 percent of the time in the CHA study and 100 percent of the time in women with fatal heart attack in the Framingham Study (61.5 percent in nonfatal heart attack). For young men, smoking was a factor 66.1 to 73.7 percent of the time in the three studies. Likewise, hypertension was present in men 73.4 percent of the time in men aged 40-59 in the CHA study and 55.5 percent in the MRFIT study. Compared with cholesterol these numbers are huge and are far above what would be expected in the general population.

It is telling that the most profound factors in creating heart disease are related to stress. People often smoke to relieve anxiety and stress, and this makes the addiction to nicotine more than just something physical. In addition, stress is known to play a role in creating most hypertension. We will discuss in later chapters just how large a role stress plays. Suffice it to say that, as the authors of this study suggested, the sole focus on cholesterol is grossly misplaced.

Summary

The risk that cholesterol levels contribute to heart disease is minimal. But, if you subscribe to the belief that cholesterol causes heart disease, then you focus on lowering your number any way possible. Drugs offer the "quick-fix," claiming to lower cholesterol almost immediately and without requiring any other intervention. By taking this route, you miss the opportunity to improve your health without pills. These improvements will affect not only your cardiovascular health, but also your overall health and well-being. Still, drugs for cholesterol have been touted for years as the most effective way to prevent heart attacks. This plays into the trap of the next myth: The Myth of the Magic Bullet.

* 5 *
THE MYTH OF THE MAGIC BULLET

---

*The belief that cholesterol medication is the solution to
heart disease.*

Leah's Story

*Leah was an office manager of a clinic when we first met her. She was
depressed and overwhelmed due to her recent divorce. She had a new job
in addition to the responsibility of her two children. Her desire to perform well was a source of intense pressure.*

*Leah was 40 pounds overweight. Her medications included drugs for
asthma, hypertension, and depression. In addition, she had been advised
to take cholesterol-lowering medication. Leah felt, however, that she
was taking enough drugs. She did not want the extra financial expense
because she understood that her cholesterol level was only mildly elevated —
210 total with an HDL of 45.*

The main reason for her visit was depression. The pharmaceutical anti-depressants were not working, so she had been taking some St. John's Wort to help her low mood. She reported some improvement with this herb, but stopped using it when her physician prescribed yet another synthetic antidepressant.

We discussed many natural approaches. Leah was encouraged to pursue the practice of meditation. She decided to learn Transcendental Meditation because of the effortless nature of this practice.

Additionally, we emphasized that she get adequate and sound sleep to stabilize her mood. We discussed strategies for handling her job stress and recommended changes in her diet. This was not a weight-loss diet, rather a nutritional plan to eliminate the buildup of toxins that had occurred over years.

Within a couple of weeks, Leah's depression had lifted. At her follow-up appointment, her blood pressure was below normal. Since she had been on two medications for blood pressure, it was suggested that she stop one of them. She was conscientious about checking her blood pressure twice daily. Leah noticed that after she stopped her first medication, her blood pressure did not change at all. In fact, it still remained lower than normal. Consequently, she was advised to wean off the last blood pressure drug. Her blood pressure remained normal in the upcoming months.

Three months later, Leah had lost 15 pounds. She was off of all medication, except for asthma drugs. Her mood had improved so much that she actually felt happy. When we rechecked her levels, her total cholesterol was 198 and her HDL was 48. Needless to say, she did not need any medication, as her risk ratio was less than 4.0.

Leah's story is significant because it is a classic case. First, it demonstrates the importance of focusing on the problem, rather than treating the symptoms. Second, it serves as evidence that the mind and body are all part of one unified system.

Without ever focusing on her cholesterol levels, we had done more to improve her heart health than would be possible with years of cholesterol-lowering medication. Undertaking the practice of meditation was healing for her heart. The fact that Leah no longer had high blood pressure eliminates a huge risk factor for heart disease. To put it in context, through meditation she was able to do naturally the equivalent of lowering her cholesterol level from 210 to 100. This is something nearly impossible to do even with powerful pharmaceutical drugs. Furthermore, her weight had dropped effortlessly. Normalizing her weight will decrease any future risk of diabetes. Since her diet had improved, so did her cholesterol levels. It is hard to believe that one effortless and natural intervention could induce such great internal changes, while simultaneously reducing stress. Meditation did more for her health than all the medication in the drug store ever could.

Relying on cholesterol-lowering medication to protect her heart would have had a negligible impact on her health in the long-term. At the core were more pressing issues like curing her hypertension, lowering her weight, and eliminating her depression. These will prove to be more effective and longer lasting interventions than taking pills for the rest of her life. This is not to mention the expense we saved her and the decreased risk of negative side effects and multiple drug interactions.

Admittedly, Leah is not the typical patient. Fortunately for her, she is willing to reject the common conditioning of the media, the pharmaceutical companies, and the medical profession. All these organizations promote the concept of "Health in a Pill." Leah was persistent in her search for answers. Moreover, she welcomed making significant changes in her lifestyle. As a result, she benefited by vastly improving her overall health. This sense of wellness can never be found in a pill.

The Magic Bullet Theory

The medical profession and the media, in particular, are fond of extolling the "miracles of modern medicine." While "miracles" do occur, more often they are more hype than reality. Nonetheless, they have reinforced the idea that the solution to most health problems comes in a pill.

This is largely a result of the style of science that has driven so many of our technological advances. This style of thinking is reductionistic. It attempts to reduce problems to a single process gone wrong. In doing so, it offers simple solutions to complex problems. In the medical field, this translates to identifying a biochemical that can manipulate the single process in a particular way.

Depression: An Example

In the case of depression, reductionistic thinking focuses on the brain's biochemicals in order to find the *cause* of this condition. Hence, depression is defined as a condition resulting from a lack of some brain substance. If this is the case, then depression should be able to be "cured" by supplying the brain with that substance. Changes in the levels of these brain biochemicals should alter mood.

By reducing complex processes to a single cause, we create the possibility of a "magic bullet." A magic bullet is one that can locate a special target in the body, hit the target and eliminate a disease all by itself. Medical history does reveal the creation of some real magic bullets. Antibiotics are a good example.

Depression, unlike some infectious diseases, is not caused by a single organism. It is an exceedingly complex condition that does not lend itself well to reductionistic thinking. Still, pharmaceutical companies have

> *Reducing complex disease processes to a single cause is often fraught with problems and side effects.*

continued to attempt to cure depression with a pill. First, they decided to look for a pill that would stimulate the brain to produce more of the "missing" biochemical. Alternatively, they looked for ways to stop its breakdown, so that higher levels could be sustained.

Serotonin is one such biochemical that has received a lot of attention. It is a neurotransmitter. (It transmits "messages" between brain cells.) The pharmacist's shelf is full of *selective serotonin reuptake inhibitors* (SSRIs). These drugs stop the metabolism of serotonin and allow brain levels of the neurotransmitter to increase.   Drugs like Prozac (fluoxetine), Paxil (paroxetine), Zoloft (sertraline), Celexa (citalopram) are all in this class.

Modern medicine's "magic bullet" has sometimes not only missed its target but has also produced devastating results. For example, it was recently found that some of these drugs may have a reverse effect on depressed teenagers. An increase in teen suicide has been associated with the use of SSRIs. This is the potential magnitude of a side effect that is created when a complex problem is oversimplified. The inner workings of the brain, let alone the mind, are yet to be fully deciphered.

Heart Disease: Another Example

Heart disease is also a complex condition. Atherosclerosis (hardening of the arteries) is the result of a very involved process. Targeting cholesterol to cure heart disease is just like targeting serotonin to cure depression. It is virtually impossible to protect the heart with such an incomplete approach and such disregard for potentially disastrous side effects. Yet, the myth of the magic bullet lives on.

Magical Mystery Tour

Our society assumes that the principles of modern medicine are based on sound research. Nowhere is this fallacy as evident as in the major studies undertaken to prove that lowering cholesterol with drugs leads to improved health. Let us take a tour of some of the most important studies.

Shocking though it may seem, the medical profession has based its recommendations for prescribing cholesterol-lowering medications on very few trials with very dubious results. How many? Six! That is correct. Only six large trials of preventing heart disease by lowering cholesterol have been undertaken to date.

These are primary prevention trials that undertake studying people who, at the onset of the trial, do not have a given disease. Their progress is then tracked for years to see if a given intervention prevented the onset of disease. Thus far, six large primary prevention trials have been published. Here is the list:

- The WHO trial, otherwise known as the World Health Organization (WHO) Cooperative Trial, which used the drug clofibrate and included 10,577 patients[1,2]

- The Bile Binding trial, cited in the literature under the name "Lipid Research Clinics Coronary Primary Prevention Trial," which utilized the drug cholestyramine (a bile acid binding medicine) and included 3,806 patients[3,4]

- The Helsinki trial, known as the Helsinki Heart Study, which utilized gemfibrozil and included 4,081 patients[5]

- The Scotland trial, otherwise known as the West of Scotland Coronary Prevention Study Group (WOSCOPS), which studied pravastatin and included 6,595 patients[6]

- The Air Force trial, officially cited as the AFCAPS/Tex-CAPS trial, which utilized lovastatin and included 6,605 patients[7]

- The Anglo-Scandinavian trial, or the ASCOT-LLA trial, which used atorvastatin and included 10,305 patients[8]

At first glance, this may appear to be a weighty volume of data supporting the importance of lowering cholesterol. However, the devil is in the details. The results of the six trials are sobering. The results of the first three trials did not show a decrease in coronary mortality. This statement is worth repeating — *no decrease in mortality from heart disease was found in these three trials*. While the studies touted a decrease in "coronary events" (nonfatal heart attacks), there were other very disturbing problems found in these studies.

What problem could be so disturbing as to offset the benefit of a lowered rate of heart attacks? The answer: An "unexpected" *increase* in overall death! Non-cardiovascular mortality increased in these three trials. That means that there was increase in death from causes other than heart disease in those taking the drugs.

Any cholesterol-lowering benefit was disturbingly overshadowed by the increase in the number of people who died while taking the drugs. Realize that, at the onset of the study, the population under investigation was presumed to be free of disease. In two studies (the WHO and Helsinki trials) cancer deaths occurred 18 to 24 percent more frequently in those receiving cholesterol-lowering drugs versus those in the control group. Total mortality (the incidence of death) increased by 25 percent in the WHO Cooperative Trial. Both of these trends were statistically significant in that study.

Let us think about this. Half of the research showed no decrease in coronary mortality. One of the three studies actually showed a negative effect (increased overall mortality). This is hardly what anyone would expect to form the scientific foundation for the billions of dollars spent each year on cholesterol drugs and cholesterol testing.

Why were there more deaths in the groups treated with cholesterol-lowering medications? Could cholesterol actually play some protective role in the body? Do these drugs create problems that result in a higher death rate? Rather than attempting to answer those questions, the cholesterol myth persisted.

> *No decrease in cardiac mortality, plus an increase in overall mortality, was found in three major trials of cholesterol medication.*

The Scotland Trial

Returning to our magical mystery tour, we are left with only three large studies to justify the popular cholesterol-phobia:

the Scotland trial, the Air Force trial and the Anglo-Scandina-vian study. The Scotland trial (WOSCOPS) was the first large-scale research to show a benefit without an immediate increase in non-cardiac mortality. But, how does this research apply to you and me? Women are out of luck, since this trial only included men. These men were between age 45 and 64 and had to have total cholesterol levels over 252 before entering the trial. In fact, the average cholesterol level was 272. Hence, as discussed in previous chapters, it is safe to assume that a good number of these subjects with such high elevations had a genetic defect in cholesterol metabolism (familial hypercholesterolemia). They are not like the average person. Even if you accept that the results are skewed and may *not* apply to the rest of us, you may still want to know the result of the study.

At the end of five years, 1.6 percent of the men in the control group and 1.2 percent of the men in the pravastatin (Prava-chol) group had died of heart disease. The difference was so small that the results were not statistically significant. If all causes of death were included, then we have the following figures: 9.4 percent had died in the control group versus 8.6 percent in the pravastatin group. This 0.8 percent benefit after five years of treatment was also not statistically signifi-cant.

The only measure that reached statistical significance was the incidence of nonfatal heart disease. This was reported as 6.2 percent in the control group and 4.3 percent in the drug treatment group. There was not even a 2 percent benefit incurred by the control group. It is only through statistical

manipulation that the trial was able to appear at all successful. (For example, they reported relative risk instead of absolute percentages).

Let us discuss this "benefit" of drug therapy another way. If
you were in the control group, your chance of living five
years without a heart attack or a heart disease-related event
was 93.8 percent. On the other hand, if you took the drug
daily for 5 years, your chances increased to 95.7 percent.
Hardly a significant enough difference to justify all the enor-
mous expense that goes into testing and manufacturing the
drugs — not to mention all the negative side effects.

Another curious aspect of the Scotland trial was the drop-out
rate. Curiously, although the results have been touted as demonstrating success, the drop-out rate was huge — 29.6 percent, or almost a third of the participants, had dropped out at
five years. Almost a third of the participants had dropped
out. Supposedly these dropouts were not related to adverse
drug effects. Subsequent analysis showed that, in those individuals with a low risk of heart disease, 66 individuals had to
be treated in order for just one person to benefit. That means
the other 65 people had no benefit whatsoever for their
efforts.

Needless to say, these numbers are sobering. The very high
starting levels of cholesterol and the lack of any female participants make it hard to understand how the results apply to

normal populations. The results are not that impressive without statistical manipulations.

SUMMARY

Three major studies showed:

    1) No impact on the number of deaths due to heart

       disease; and

    2) An increase in all-cause deaths when elevated

       cholesterol is treated with drugs.

The other study showed a minimal benefit in a group that likely included a number of people with a genetic defect in cholesterol metabolism.

Only two major trials are left to solve the magical mystery of why the medical community has claimed firm scientific footing for lowering cholesterol with drugs in people without heart disease.

The Air Force Trial (AFCAPS/TexCAPS)

The Air Force trial was a randomized, placebo-controlled trial testing the use of 20 to 40 mg daily of lovastatin in patients without heart disease. It differed from the Scotland trial in two major ways. First, 997 postmenopausal women were included. Second, the mean total serum cholesterol was

221 mg/dL and the LDL-cholesterol averaged 150 mg/dL. These numbers are much closer to the averages in the normal population and would likely represent fewer individual with familial hypercholesterolemia.

After 5.2 years, the absolute benefit was 2 percent. In other words, treating 1000 individuals resulted in 19 fewer "coronary events," of which 12 were heart attacks. What about mortality rates? The mortality rate in the treatment group was 2.4 percent and in the control group 2.3 percent. Yes, that is correct: The death rate was less in the control group, but the difference was not statistically significant. Thus, from this study we observe no difference in death rates and a mere 2 percent absolute benefit after 5.2 years of therapy. Would it raise your suspicion to know that co-workers of three of the lead study organizers were employees of Merck?[9] Merck is the pharmaceutical company that makes lovastatin and markets it as Mevacor. Perhaps this explains why the results may have been presented in glowing fashion as "proof" that treating cholesterol makes a big difference in preventing heart disease.

Onc has to wonder, though, why the difference in heart attack rates did not result in a difference in death rates. Was something in the drug making death from heart attack more likely? In other words, even if there were fewer heart attacks, more of them were fatal. Either way an absolute benefit of 2 percent and a 0 percent benefit in preventing death is hardly the basis to guide all of our preventive strategies. Perhaps our final study will be so extraordinarily impressive as to compensate all the others' weak results.

The Anglo-Scandinavian Trial (ASCOT-LLA)

The Anglo-Scandinavian trial evaluated 19,342 hypertensive individuals randomized to one of two blood pressure treatments. The lipid-lowering part of this trial randomly assigned 10,305 patients with cholesterol of 251 or less to treatment with atorvastatin or placebo. But wait. This is a study of people with high blood pressure. What if people with hypertension react differently to medication than those with just high cholesterol? This is another example of the misapplication of the results of a study to the average person. Generalizing from such a study to a population without hypertension is fraught with potential errors. So our final study has not solved the mystery.

> *It remains a mystery why the medical profession feels so confident in utilizing cholesterol-lowering drugs for primary prevention.*

The essence of the cholesterol myth is that by lowering cholesterol you can prevent heart disease and save lives without creating ill health. This was not the case in the first three studies, and the subsequent two showed almost no impact on mortality at all.

Still, what was the impact of the cholesterol-lowering medication on the people with high blood pressure in the ASCOT-LLA trial? As stated in the article: "The study did not show statistically significant reductions in all-cause mortality or cardiovascular mortality." In addition, subgroups with different starting levels of total cholesterol seemed to have similar relative risk reductions in terms of non-fatal heart attack and coronary heart disease. In essence, regardless of the initial cholesterol level, the drug helped a bit.

This does not fit the cholesterol theory. Only those with high cholesterol should be helped, not everyone across the board. Clearly, the drug's positive affect then is not due to lowering cholesterol. Is the drug exerting its effect in another way?

It remains a mystery why the medical profession feels so confident in utilizing cholesterol-lowering drugs for primary prevention given the paucity of data in those without pre-existing heart disease. If cholesterol *caused* heart disease, then certainly lowering it should show dramatic decreases in death from heart attack. The absolute decreases in heart disease should be large. In addition, the incidence of heart disease should directly correlate with elevations in cholesterol. But data from these studies are not impressive. It does not lend any concrete support to the theory that cholesterol causes heart disease. In fact, in some instances it appears to prove exactly the opposite.

A Landmark Study

The Scandinavian Simvastatin Survival Study (4S) is considered a landmark study of cholesterol-lowering in patients with coronary heart disease.[12,13,14] It reported a "significant" reduction in heart attack, stroke, and death. It thereby put to rest the concern created by earlier studies that cholesterol-lowering would increase overall mortality, even if it reduced heart disease. This study formed the basis for much of the treatment strategy of utilizing "statin" drugs in modern cardiology. Statin drugs are those like Lipitor (atorvastatin), Mevacor (lovastatin), and Zocor (simvastatin) that block the synthesis of cholesterol in the body.

> *159 people had to be treated with simvastatin for a year in order to prevent just one cardiac event.*

Let us take a closer look at the data. How great was the absolute reduction in death? The results showed a 3.3 percent reduction in mortality over 5.4 years. If we look at relative risk it appears huge — 29 percent. However, when viewed from the perspective of the number needed to treat, this figure loses its luster. One hundred fifty-nine individuals had to be treated with the drug for a year to prevent just one of them from having a cardiac event. But, unlike previous studies, these results at least point to some benefit gained by people with known heart disease. This is not, however, the end of the story.

The LIPID Study: Not the Fat-Lowering Effect after All

Another landmark trial was the LIPID study. [15] This study included 9,014 men and women who had a recent heart attack or suffered from chest pain upon physical exertion (unstable angina). Participants were given either pravastatin (Pravachol) or placebo. The study outcomes were similar to the 4S study, demonstrating only a 3 percent reduction in mortality.

Yet, something interesting also occurred. The drug seemed to benefit even those with low cholesterol levels. In fact, the benefit of pravastatin was seen across the board in all age subgroups. It occurred irrespective of the serum concentration of total cholesterol, LDL-cholesterol, HDL-cholesterol or triglycerides. A benefit was also incurred by individuals with higher cholesterol levels, increased age, smokers, and those who had a heart attack. How could this be explained?

The LIPID study provided evidence to what scientists were already beginning to suspect — the statins helped by means other than lowering cholesterol. Certainly, this had to be the case if people with *low* cholesterol also benefited from the drug. This suspicion had been raised by studies showing plaque regression after only six months of drug therapy when it was known that it took almost two years to get a significant change in atherosclerosis with cholesterol reduction.

While some studies such as the Heart Protection Study[16] showed only a 1.8 percent reduction in mortality, other studies have shown no reduction, such as the MIRACL trial of atorvastatin (Lipitor).[17] The MIRACL trial showed that atorvastatin did not prevent death, heart attack, or the need for revascularization (heart bypass surgery). Most people never hear about the *lack* of positive findings in some studies.

Overall, these clinical trials showed a small benefit incurred by using statin drugs. Most people are shocked by how minimal the benefit is when considered in context. Remember that these benefits occur in individuals who already have heart disease, not in those without it. Below is a table summarizing the results.

Trials of Statin Drugs in Patients with Known Heart Disease

Study Name	Subjects	Absolute Reduction in Mortality	Mortality Relative Risk Reduction	Absolute Reduction in Heart Attacks (Cardiac Events)	Relative Risk Reduction in Heart Attacks (Cardiac Events)
4S	4,444	3.3%	29%	6.7%	30%
LIPID	9,014	3.0%	21%	2.9%	27%
Heart Protection Study	20,536	1.8%	13%	5.4%	24%
MIRACL	3,086	0%	0%	2.6%	16%
AVERAGE		**2.0%**	**16%**	**4.4%**	**24%**

The benefits derived from statin use are most likely not related to their cholesterol-lowering effects. In fact, cholesterol-lowering may be just a "side effect" of this class of drugs. The statin drugs are now known to do other things:

1) Cause an increase in the number of more buoyant LDL particles, which are thought to be less damaging to arteries; and
2) Increase the resistance of cholesterol to oxidation.

Both of these mechanisms will result in decreased plaque formation. In light of this information, what can we surmise about the way statin drugs exert their effect?

Statins — An Expensive Aspirin by Any Other Name

Statins work. The research shown unequivocally, albeit minimally, that they reduce the risk of heart attacks in people with heart disease. Why?

We have determined that statin drugs do not simply lower the cholesterol levels in the blood. Often it takes two years to see significant reversal of atherosclerosis when cholesterol levels are lowered. Yet, curiously enough, the studies on statins show an immediate reduction in heart attack rates.

This surprising finding fascinated research scientists. Upon further investigation, it was revealed that statins interfere with the clotting process in the body. They affect the function of fibrinogen thereby reducing the risk of clot formation, much like aspirin does (but by a different mechanism). Thus, the immediate reduction in heart attacks is not due to the cholesterol-lowering effects of the statins. Although this hypothesis has not been directly tested, statins may just be a very expensive form of aspirin.

Recent studies have prompted cardiologists to recommend that people who have coronary artery disease be placed on statins *regardless* of their cholesterol levels. Again, statins are effective in reducing the risk of heart attacks because they interrupt clot formation, not because they lower cholesterol levels in the blood. From a logical perspective, taking these drugs should only be recommended if there is a high risk of heart attack.

Efficacy of Statins

And then, how good are these drugs? This is the other problem with the magic bullet theory. Statins do not work like antibiotics. They don't "cure" heart disease by eliminating the offending party. They are less than 100 percent effective. From the table above, it is clear that most studies have similar results and show a relative risk reduction of approximately 24 percent. In absolute terms the numbers are typically very small — 1 to 3 percent. *Note: Keep this value in the forefront of your mind — 24 percent risk reduction. We will use this number for comparisons in later chapters.*

Consider what this means in terms of the number needed to treat. We typically have to put as many as 125 individuals on statins to help just one of them. The other 124 receive no benefit whatsoever.

A 24 percent risk reduction means that a lot of heart attacks occur *in spite of being on the drug*. To illustrate this point, let us assume that 100 heart attacks are expected to occur in a given group of people. If, instead, they take the drug, then, based on these numbers, 24 fewer heart attacks would occur. Still,

76 taking the drug would suffer a heart attack. Drug treatment failed to protect almost three-fourths of the people.

This is sobering news for anyone who holds out hope for a magic bullet solution. It does not prevent the majority of heart attacks from occurring. In fact, many of the people taking the statins will have heart attacks anyway. Add to this scenario the costs of treatment, testing, and harmful side effects. The question remains: Is the mythical gamble worth the cost?

Statins — Perhaps an Expensive Vitamin?

Scientists now know that statin drugs also exert an antioxidant effect. Recall that the antioxidant drug, probucol, caused a reversal of their heart disease in rabbits. Statins have free-radical scavenging abilities. This is the more likely explanation of how they reverse atherosclerosis. Free radicals damage the endothelial cells. This is the initiating step in the process of plaque formation. Moreover, free radicals abound when cholesterol is oxidized in macrophages. If there are no free radicals and the oxidation process ceases, then the process of atherosclerosis stops. In plaques that are not old and calcified, healing of the inflamed areas probably causes disease reversal.

Perhaps statins are just an expensive vitamin. As we will see in Chapter 7, a more effective way to introduce the protective effect of antioxidants is through diet by eating fruits and vegetables rich in vitamins E and C. (Maybe Mom was right!)

Sam's Story: Don't Judge a Book by its Cover

The problem with the magic bullet theory of cholesterol drugs is that it gives people a false sense of security. It distracts people from realizing that heart disease is a complex process and that the most important ways of preventing it do not involve cholesterol management. Consider Sam's story.

Sam came to our clinic after having a minor heart attack and triple bypass surgery. Three of the main vessels supplying blood to the heart were "clogged" by plaques, so veins were taken from his legs to "bypass" (re-route) the blood over the clogged areas.

Sam was chronically sleep-deprived. He was using caffeine to keep himself functional. His life had become extremely stressful. Facing debt, he tried to compensate by working extra hours. His life was complicated with raising his children and his wife's children from a former marriage.

Prior to this heart attack, Sam had subsided on an all-American diet of daily fast food for lunch. Lunch was his main meal. During afternoons and evenings, he filled himself with snacks, particularly potato chips. In spite of this, Sam's thin frame did not accumulate weight. Sam considered himself "lucky" to be able to eat the greasy, fatty foods he loved without gaining weight.

After his surgery, he was put on three drugs, two for his heart and one for his cholesterol. He had difficulty tolerating the medications. One medication caused such an intense drop in blood pressure that he felt like he was about to pass out every time he stood up. Still, he continued to take his cholesterol medication.

He came to us over a year later because he was starting to experience chest pain: "I don't know why I am having this. The bypass grafts can't be clogged already, can they? My cholesterol is 40 points lower than before."

We discussed his dietary habits and the stresses in his life. In the year since his surgery, little had changed in this regard. In fact, his financial worries were even greater because of potential layoffs at his company. I recommended he undergo further testing with his cardiologist to see if his grafts were clogged. In fact, this was the case.

Sam had been under the illusion that drugs had cured him. His cholesterol level was lower than average, and his blood pressure was low thanks to the drugs. He thought he would never have problems with atherosclerosis again.

This is precisely the problem with the magic bullet approach. It deceives people into thinking they are safe or cured, while, unfortunately, the disease process continues on. It keeps people from focusing on important changes in dietary, emotional, and mental patterns that are the main causes of heart disease.

Sam eventually returned for advice on how he could reverse his atherosclerosis after having another medical procedure to unclog one of his arteries. He was ready to radically change his dietary habits and address the stress in his life. Two years later, his arteries showed a slight improvement. More importantly, they did not continue to clog. Getting rid of his reliance on a magic bullet made all the difference.

The Hidden Costs of Drug Therapy

When magic bullets like antibiotics are prescribed, the instructions never read: Take this pill for the "rest of your life." After all, the idea is that it eradicates the offender quickly, efficiently, and forever. It cures the illness without negative side effects. Therein lies the magic.

Long-term drug use is a giant experiment on the human race without long-term data. Never before in the history of the human species has the body been subjected to chemical drugs, year in, year out. While the Food and Drug Administration has set up an elaborate system for trying to test the safety and efficacy of new drugs, never have they required lengthy long-term studies to be completed on any medication. It is all too often that after a drug is released, disastrous side effects come to light. Then, the drug is pulled from the market.

One such drug already mentioned is Baycol. This cholesterol-lowering medication was approved by the FDA and became widely used. It was not until it had been on the market for almost three years that the FDA became aware of problems that demanded they reverse their approval. A number of people developed destruction of muscle tissue which overwhelmed the body and caused death. This condition is known as rhabdomyolysis and had occurred in rare cases with some other statin drugs. But the occurrence of several deaths within a short time prompted review of the drug. It was then pulled off the market.

The recent history of the FDA is plagued with other similar stories. Various media sources have hyped the wonders of modern medicine. This has played into this myth of the magic bullet promoted by modern science. Our society has been bombarded by the message that popping a pill can solve complex problems. Not until faced with dire consequences do we want to take a serious look at other offending factors — namely, our lifestyle and habits.

The list of recent drug failures continues to grow with the Vioxx scandal creating a huge wave of lawsuits in late 2004. The result is that one cannot help but question a system that bases recommendations for prevention on flimsy evidence without ample drug testing. In many ways, the craving for a quick fix, for "health in a pill," has created the largest population of guinea pigs in the world. With minimal testing and little monitoring of the pharmaceutical industry, the current drug culture is truly a giant experiment. We wait with anticipation to see what potential side effects may arise from ingesting chemicals that stimulate limited biological processes. The list of "experimental failures" is lengthy.

Critical Condition

An excellent portrayal of the state of the American health care system can be found in a book by Donald L. Barlett and James B. Steele called *Critical Condition*. They describe how health care has become "big business" and how this has led to "bad" medicine. In describing the role of the media in the demise of health care, they note how the media has tended to exaggerate the efficacy of new drugs and ignore their side effects. They catalog some of the colossal failures of modern drugs in support of their view. In addition to the previously mentioned Baycol, they describe other medicines that have been approved by the FDA only to later be found to cause problems. These include:

- Rezulin, introduced in 1977, was in a new class of drugs touted to revolutionize the care of Type II diabetes. Three years later, the drug was pulled from the market because it caused liver failure — many patients had died, and others required liver transplants.

- Bextra, a drug initially used for arthritis pain and menstrual cramps that was later promoted for all types of pain in adults, was initially approved in November 2001. The drug company was later forced to amend its label when some patients developed "life-threatening" complications.

- Posicor, a blood pressure medication, was taken off the market in 1998 because it was lethal when taken with more than two dozen other medicines.

- Lotronex, a treatment for irritable bowel syndrome, was taken off the market the same year it was introduced — 2000. It caused colitis, intestinal damage, and ruptured bowels.

- Seldane, a treatment for seasonal allergies, was taken off the market in 1997 because it caused serious and sometimes fatal cardiac arrhythmias.

- Propulsid, a treatment for reflux disease and heartburn, was linked to cardiac arrhythmias in 300 patients, 80 of whom died.

Putting faith in the power of magic bullets can be deadly. Moving away from a "pill-popping" mentality toward a culture of self-care and lifestyle awareness is the shift that is needed in medicine today. Without it, the magic bullet approach will only continue to predominate, with the mirage of promoting health and its illusion of safety. What we need is a deeper understanding of what causes heart disease and what creates heart health.

SECTION II:
CREATING HEART HEALTH

* 6 *
MIND OVER MATTER

The Real Killer

What if you don't have many risk factors for heart disease? Then, measuring cholesterol is of little use. Large decreases in your cholesterol levels may only yield a 1 to 2 percent reduction in your five-year risk of heart disease. That is the bottom line.

Are there other factors that are important? As mentioned before, anything that can create microscopic injury in blood vessels is a risk factor. Although medical science has attempted to characterize these factors, one risk factor is yet to be fully appreciated by the medical community.

This risk factor is alluded to by one of the quiz questions given in our Preventive Medicine Seminar. Below is the question:

> *When do most heart attacks occur?*
> *A. At night*
> *B. At noon*
> *C. Monday morning at 9 A.M.*
> *D. No specific time*

The body has an internal clock. This is the basis for so-called biorhythms, which seem to be organized around light and dark cycles. However, the body has no mechanism for knowing the day of the week (i.e. Monday from Tuesday or Saturday). Yet most heart attacks in the United States occur Monday at 9 A.M. Something is triggering heart-attacks that is not related to biorhythms or physical processes.

> *It is stress that is triggering heart attacks, not cholesterol.*

In the United States, the vast majority of people do not like their jobs. They usually have the weekend off and then must return to a stressful work environment that is unfulfilling. It is stress that is triggering heart attacks, not cholesterol. Stress is killing people.

Stress is a much underrated factor in heart health. Unlike cholesterol, it cannot be measured directly or quantified easily. It cannot be examined under a microscope. Hence, it is marginalized to the realm of the nonphysical.

The Look of Stress

Stress plays a huge role in creating physical disease. Hans Selye is considered the father of modern stress research. As was the case with most medical training programs, Selye's first exposure to patients was in a large amphitheater. A patient with a certain disease was led into the front stage of an amphitheater filled with medical students. Questions about symptoms were tossed around; signs of disease pointed out. In this manner, students learned firsthand how each disease appears different from the next.

> *Stress is a much under-rated factor in heart health.*

Selye was not, however, the typical medical student. Most were simply intent on memorizing the characteristic features of each disease and evaluating the presentation of each patient for these classical signs and symptoms. Selye was curious about what he was seeing. While he noticed the differences in each patient, what surprised him was a simple observation: "They all *looked* sick."

He began wondering what was causing this "sick look." What was it about every illness that made each patient obviously look unwell? Selye thought there was something unifying about all illness. This was the beginning of his formulation of the theory of stress.

Selye began to wonder if there were other ways in which this ill condition could be induced without giving an animal or a person a disease. He found that putting animals under stressful conditions produced similar changes. What were some of these changes?

Putting his laboratory animals under stress caused them to age more quickly. They began to "look" older. This seems to be the case with humans who are ill, as well. They had elevated levels of cortisol and norepinephrine in the bloodstream. If they weren't starved, they tended to accumulate fatty tissue in the abdomen. Their adrenal glands tended to enlarge. And, they tended to get atherosclerosis.

Stress on the Heart

Stress is known to play a role in creating both atherosclerosis and heart attack. While some of the mechanisms still need to be elucidated, it is clear that stress elevates blood levels of adrenaline-like substances called catecholamines. Higher levels of catecholamines are known to alter the function of macrophages. These immune cells are responsible for recruiting cholesterol into plaques. More specifically, when macrophages are stimulated by catecholamine, they produce more oxidized cholesterol particles. As you may recall, oxidized cholesterol is responsible for damaging the cells lining the artery.

In addition, blood levels of cholesterol have been shown to rise during stressful situations.[1,2,3] The increases in blood cholesterol range from 8 to 65 percent in situations such as the preparation of tax returns in April by accountants, the taking of examinations by students, and following job loss or significant life events.[4] The mechanism by which this rise occurs is yet unclear. It is postulated that it may result from the release of fat from cells when they are triggered by adrenaline-like substances (catecholamines).[5]

Stress has a direct physical impact on the cardiovascular system in other ways. Studies have shown the following:

- **Blood Vessel Injury:** In animal studies, psychological stress produces endothelial injury perhaps via the activation of neurohormonal and hormonal substances. [6,7,8] For example, emotional agitation creates blood turbulence, which, in turn, injures arteries, particularly at branch points. Recall that injury to the endothelium is the first step in the generation of atherosclerosis. Damage to the endothelium will promote the following: movement of lipoproteins from the circulation to the artery wall, platelet aggregation, and the release of growth factors that cause scar formation.

- **Blood Vessel Dysfunction:** A brief period of mental stress can cause transient endothelial dysfunction in young healthy individuals without evidence of vascular disease or risk factors for cardiovascular disease. The level of mental stress described in studies is unlike that occurring in everyday life. [9,10] The endothelial dysfunction lasts for as long as one to four hours.[11,12] Also, during mental stress, the blood vessels of individuals with high blood pressure, but not high cholesterol, do not expand appropriately in response to potent biochemicals that cause arteries to dilate, such as nitric oxide.[13]

- **Clot Formation:** Mental stress and increased exposure to epinephrine can lead to platelet activation and deposition.[14,15.,16] This is the beginning of clot formation in the arteries.

- **Triggers Other Injurious Behaviors:** Psychosocial factors may also promote atherosclerosis via an effect on other risk factors. For example, cigarette smokers typically increase their consumption of cigarettes in response to stress. Among others, cigarette smoke loads the body with damaging free radicals, which, in turn, damage arterial walls.

Stress and hypertension are thought to be related. As we saw in Chapter 4, hypertension is a very potent risk factor for heart disease. It towers over cholesterol in importance.

There is a strong correlation between high blood pressure and psychosocial variables of a stressful nature, such as job loss and demanding occupations. Animal studies provide even more compelling evidence for sustained hypertension resulting from emotional stress.[17] Although an increase in blood pressure in response to stress is well described in humans, the change tends to return to normal following removal of the stress.[18] However, a more prolonged response may be seen in those with a genetic predisposition to hypertension. As an example, individuals with a family history of high blood pressure show exaggerated cardiovascular responsiveness to stressors when compared to those without a family history of hypertension. Furthermore, hyperreactivity may be a marker for individuals at increased risk for developing hypertension. The mechanism behind the rise in blood pressure may be related to increased blood levels of catecholamines.

Burning the Heart with Anger

Surrogate markers for stress are also known to play a significant role in heart attack. Anger is one such marker. Anger in response to stress may be of particular importance for the development of premature cardiovascular disease in young men.

This issue was addressed in a longitudinal study of 1,055 male medical students. They were asked to report anger reactions to stress on a questionnaire.[19] Thirty-six years later, those with the highest self-reported level of anger had a statistically significant increased risk of premature cardiovascular disease. That is, they developed heart disease before the age of 55.

How significant was the impact of anger on heart disease? Recall from the previous chapter that drugs could offer a reduction in risk in the range of 24 percent. Within this context, let us appreciate the impact of having low and high anger reactions to stress on health status. The decrease in relative risk in those with lower levels of anger was 210 percent less (relative risk 3.1). Now, if becoming calm and less angry were a drug, it would cause this effect: a *210 percent* decrease in risk of premature coronary heart disease, a *250 percent* decreased risk of coronary heart disease (relative risk 3.5), and a decrease in myocardial infarction of *540 percent* (relative risk 6.4).

You can see now why the drug's influence is paltry compared to stress reduction. By taking a drug you can lower your relative risk by 24 percent. Alternatively, you can learn to reduce stress in your life and reduce your risk by over 210 percent. Allow us to put this in perspective with a graphic illustration:

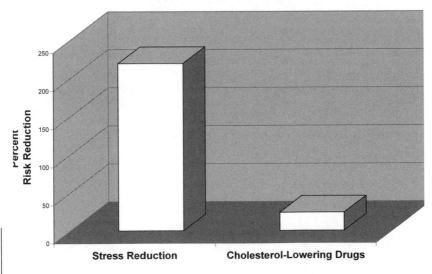

You choose which makes the most sense to focus your time, effort, money, and energy pursuing.

The Finland Study

Another study that supports the overwhelming importance of stress was undertaken in Finland. A study of 812 factory workers evaluated work stress with a self-assessment questionnaire.[20] After 26 years, 73 subjects (9 percent) died of cardiovascular causes. Employees with high levels of work stress had a higher cardiovascular mortality than those with lower levels of work stress. How much higher? One hundred twenty percent. Again compared with the 24 percent relative risk reductions seen in drug trials, the reduction in risk seen in those workers with lower levels of stress was huge — 120 percent (relative risk of 2.2) for an index of "job strain."

> *Those with the highest level of depression, anger, or social competitiveness had an increased risk of coronary heart disease.*

The Normative Aging Study

In a related study, the importance of personality variables showed how psychological factors can play a major role in heart disease. The Normative Aging Study followed 1,305 men of a mean age of 62 who were free of coronary heart disease.[21] After a mean follow-up of seven to eight years, those with the highest level of depression, anger, or social competitiveness (dominance) on psychological testing had an increased risk of coronary heart disease. This included nonfatal infarction and coronary death. Compared to those with the lowest levels of these traits, the increase risk due to high levels of depression, anger, and social competitiveness was 46 percent, 215 percent, and 80 percent, respectively.[22,23,24]

> *Stress and psychological factors play a huge role in heart disease.*

Stress and psychological factors play a huge role. Compared with drug therapy, stress reduction interventions shows large gains. Unfortunately, without research funding from large pharmaceutical companies, there is limited large-scale research on stress reduction as an intervention to reduce heart disease. But, there have been a few studies that are very telling.

Lost in the Counterculture

Stress was just an interesting academic subject in the late 1950s and early 1960s. At that point, there did not seem to be much to do about it. Just like catching a cold, it was generally accepted that stress would creep into each person's life at some point. But, slowly the correlates of stress in the human physiology had begun to be characterized.

It became known that under stress, the following physiologic changes occur:

- Blood pressure increases;

- Cortisol levels increase;

- Galvanic skin resistance tends to go down; and,

- Plasma lactate levels tend to go up.

Some researchers had also noticed a correlation between stress and the development of certain diseases. But, it was not until the late 1960s that some innovative research demonstrated that the mind could actually influence the body.

The body-mind connection was not an accepted concept during this time. From our current vantage point, it is difficult to imagine resistance to accepting this notion. Likewise it is now hard to imagine what it would be like to live in the 1500s when the cultural belief held that the world was flat. The point is that the scientific environment of the early 1960s was different compared to today.

Stress was not a common word. The body was thought to be essentially separate from the mind. Biofeedback was in its infancy. Biofeedback researchers were challenging a long-held belief that the autonomic nervous system was outside of conscious control. Inherent in its name — autonomic — the belief was that the body's functions were automatic. Extensive biofeedback research was needed to convince biologist, physiologists, and medical scientists otherwise. Eventually, though, this research demonstrated that body temperature, skin resistance, and even the production of stress hormones like cortisol and norepinephrine could be altered consciously with adequate biofeedback training.

This opened the minds of academics to the notion that perhaps something could be done to counter the effects of stress. The time was ripe for the introduction of meditation in the quickly changing culture of the late 1960s. Meditation was an antidote to stress. By the early '70s, this notion became so widespread that society in general began to understand the concept of stress, and millions of Americans began the practice of meditation.

This was fortunate for Harvard graduate student Robert Keith Wallace. He was able to obtain subjects for an experiment to prove that meditation could affect physiological functioning in a manner that did not involve biofeedback instruction. In conjunction with Herbert Benson, he proved that meditation could lower stress using measurement parameters such as cortisol levels, plasma lactate levels, and blood pressure. His research was later published in *Scientific American* in 1972. This work was based on the scientific technique of Transcendental Meditation. Unfortunately, this aspect of the research got relegated to the area of the counterculture, and Transcendental Meditation never became part of allopathic medicine's armamentarium.

Meditation as Medication

What if Robert Keith Wallace's research had stimulated a flood of cardiovascular research, and the medical profession had started prescribing and conducting large scale studies regarding the impact of meditation on health? In addition to seeing the impact of stress reduction on health in general, specific measures of cardiovascular disease could have been obtained. We would have had a more concrete measure of the impact and role that stress plays in cardiovascular disease and in its prevention. Perhaps there would have been large pools of people practicing meditation. A group so large, in fact, that we could look at their insurance utilization and get a good sense of the impact meditation had on their health.

As luck would have it, we do not have to wait for the next counterculture revolution in order to do this kind of study. In the 1970s and 1980s, a college was founded for people interested in gaining traditional academic degrees in an environment where all of the faculty, students, and staff practiced Transcendental Meditation (TM). The college is called Maharishi International University. Like most colleges of the time, it offered health insurance to its faculty and staff. In addition, though, it offered health insurance to those who practiced Transcendental Meditation who did not live on the campus. This plan was administered through a major insurance carrier in the state of Iowa and included more than 2,000 members.

With this fortuitous situation, a research study could be done to compare the impact of practicing TM on health. A researcher named David Orme-Johnson was able to compare the meditators to the insurer's other 600,000 members in terms of medical care and charges (both inpatient and outpatient) over a period of five years. To control for the effects of age on the results, health-care utilization was analyzed for three age categories: 0-18, 19-39, and 40-plus years. The average level of health care expenditures as well as number of medical and surgical hospital admissions were assessed for individuals during the five-year period of the study. These were then categorized in terms of type of disorder — for example, mental disorders, pregnancy and childbirth, or infectious disease. Of particular interest was one study category: heart and blood vessels. To account for any influence of self-selection, the study compared subgroups from the large number of non-meditating members in terms of professional membership, size of group, age, insurance terms, and gender.

> *The meditators had 87.3 percent less health care expenditures for cardiovascular disease.*

The results of the study were profound. Even though the TM group's demographics were similar when compared to the non-meditating groups, the number of days of hospitalization varied dramatically. For children up to age 18, it was 50.2 percent less. This was also the case for those 19 to 39 years of age. For older adults (age 40 and over), the reduction in inpatient days was 69.4 percent less. Outpatient visits for the three groups were also dramatically less: 46.8, 54.7, and 73.7 percent, for the respective age-groups.

When looking at 17 major categories of disease, the TM group had an average of 55.4 percent less admissions for benign and malignant tumors, 30.4 percent less for all infectious diseases, 30.6 percent less for mental disorders, and 87.3 percent less for heart disease.[25] Even the most powerful medications don't have the power to reduce hospital admissions by 87 percent. This is greater than triple the effect of even the best cholesterol-lowering drug trials. Moreover, it represents an *absolute* reduction in cardiovascular disease.

Research evaluators are quick to point out weaknesses in the analysis. One such problem is that the control group (non-meditators) was selected after the fact. The only way to be sure that one is not comparing apples and oranges is to identically match each meditator with a non-meditator with the exact same health history, family history, and risk profile. This seemed an impossibility until researcher Robert Herron entered the picture.

Herron's idea was this: Why not use each meditator as his or her own control? That way we know for sure that we have an identical match. How did he do this?

Fortunately for Herron, our neighbors to the north have a national system of health care. In Canada, the utilization of health care resources can be tracked on an individual basis. Herron was able to obtain data on Canadian practitioners of Transcendental Meditation. His information covered six years in total, including three years before and after initiating the practice of meditation. Then, one can confidently extrapolate what the reduction in health-care utilization would be at five years out. A consistent figure can be found.

This study confirmed Orme-Johnson's findings. Meditators had approximately a 50 percent reduction in health care utilization.[26] He later found an even greater reduction in the population over 65 years of age[27]

These numbers are "hard data" in that they concretely demonstrate the power of meditation. However, this is not the "hard science" that most medical researchers like to see. They like to randomly assign participants into a treatment or a placebo group. This is to ensure that the groups are equal and that any effect is truly due to the intervention.

To this effect, the National Institutes of Health (NIH) has spent more than 21 million dollars on research on Transcendental Meditation. Most of this research has been in high-risk minority populations. Robert Schneider, M.D., undertook a study of blood pressure reduction in African-Americans living in Oakland, California.[28,29] Individuals with elevated blood pressure were assigned either to learn the technique of Transcendental Meditation or to a standard educational program on diet and lifestyle. The results proved conclusively that meditation lowered blood pressure. Moreover, meditation caused a reduction in blood pressure equivalent to reductions seen when patients begin taking blood pressure medications.

> *The TM group had a 97.1 percent compliance rate at 3 months.*

The last point is of interest considering that compliance with blood pressure-lowering medication is notoriously low. These drugs often have negative side effects. Also, no one wants to be on medication for the rest of their lives. Most health-care providers hesitate recommending nondrug therapies because they doubt that people will do them. Schneider's study, however, showed that the TM group had a

97.1 percent compliance rate at three months after initial instruction. This is unheard of for even the best of drug strategies. The participants found meditation to be so enjoyable that the practice was easy to cultivate. That a high-risk inner-city population could benefit by a nonpharmacological means with 97 percent compliance was indeed profound news.

Hypertension is a huge risk factor for cardiovascular disease. It poses a much greater risk than cholesterol. Some studies have even shown it to be more detrimental than smoking. The practice of TM was offering a nonpharmacological way to reverse one of the main contributors to heart disease. Additionally, research on Transcendental Meditation has also shown impact on two other factors: smoking and aging. Students report "dropping" the habit of smoking after learning the technique. Other research has shown that it appears to *reverse* biological aging. Biological measures of aging, such as near-point vision, hearing acuity, and blood pressure tend to improve with meditation, suggesting that aging is actually reversed. Remember that aging is one of the most significant risk factors for heart disease.

The only criticism of these studies is that they had a relatively small number of participants. Otherwise, the study design reflected hard-core science. It was a prospective study that utilized a randomized population with a control group. Moreover, the study involved a population known for its high incidence of cardiovascular disease and its difficulty with accessing health care due to poverty and a lack of education. The studies were rigorous enough to be published in some of the most prestigious medical journals.

Another interesting study undertaken by Schneider and Nidich was to look at the oxidation of lipids in people who meditate. They measured lipid peroxide levels and found that, after controlling for dietary factors and smoking, those who meditated had 15 percent lower levels of lipid peroxides (i.e., lipoproteins damaged by free radicals).[30]

> *Stress is a huge killer. It towers over cholesterol in importance.*

Stress is a huge killer. It towers over cholesterol in importance. It has been an elusive factor because it is difficult to test and monitor. Also, stress has been accepted as part of life. The pervasive attitude is that little can be done to minimize its impact. Here, finally, was conclusive evidence that stress has a solution.

The research on Transcendental Meditation has proven that there is an answer to stress. The solution is natural and with no negative side effects. Moreover, it involves an enjoyable and effortless process.

Why Meditation Works

Meditation reduces stress by providing a deep, restful state that has been described as "hypo-metabolic." This means that there is a decrease in both respiratory and pulse rates.

Oxygen consumption decreases to levels below that of the deepest sleep. During this state, the biochemistry of the body is dramatically altered. The production of stress hormones is dramatically reduced. The body produces less cortisol and less adrenaline-like substances. Blood levels of lactate decrease. Lactate levels are measured as a surrogate marker for anaerobic stress. Blood pressure decreases 5 to 10mm systolic. Lastly, the galvanic skin response (a stress measure of skin moisture) improves. Some studies also report decreased levels of blood cholesterol. This hypo-metabolic state gives the body deep rest. It reflects the state of inner peace that the mind experiences.

This deep rest is restorative in and of itself. But, the effects of meditation carry over into the day. Decreased stress and improved rest helps all kinds of different functions. Studies have shown improvements in the following: memory, IQ, and learning ability. It also positively affects self-confidence and the ability to relate well to others. Creativity is shown to increase, and productivity in the workplace is enhanced.

Other forms of meditation have also shown reductions in stress-related variables. However, with regard to cardiovascular variables, not all meditation forms are alike. Research indicates that Transcendental Meditation may be more efficacious.[31] Still, in general, practicing some form of meditation is better than doing nothing at all. Clearly, doing whatever you can to decrease stress and increase happiness will be beneficial to your heart.

Creating a Healthier Heart

Stress is much more influential than cholesterol in creating heart disease. Stress has an antidote — meditation. It is our number one recommendation in terms of protecting the heart and producing overall health. There are also other recommendations. Here is a more detailed list:

- **Meditation** — Overwhelmingly important in creating heart health, as previously discussed. See the Resources section at the end of the book for information on how to learn the technique of Transcendental Meditation. One cannot effectively learn the technique by reading a book. In order to get the maximum benefit from meditation, a teacher is required.

- **Decrease Overcommitment** — This applies to all areas of life. Americans tend to overwork, overplay, and spend excessively. All this results in exhaustion. Overcommitment creates burdens. Similar to a horse trying to pull a 10-ton truck, exhaustion and fatigue quickly ensue. Evaluate what you have taken on and determine what groups, committees, organizations, and regular outings are really necessary. In addition, avoid debt as much as possible. Much financial stress results from the assumption that income will always be the same or that you can "put up" with the same job for a few more years. When the job scene starts to shift, a heavy debt-burden can create huge anxiety and stress.

- **Decrease Overscheduling** — If every minute of the day is scheduled, you will never be able to relax and let down. An accentuated sense of time and living by the clock creates unnecessary stress. If you must schedule everything, then also schedule downtime when you can relax or take a break in the day. Schedule in fun-time, as well. Put the tennis game in the schedule. Make an appointment with your loved ones. As much as possible, thin out the schedule to only that which must absolutely get done. You will find that most of it can wait. *Think for a moment what would be a reasonable schedule if you were recovering from a heart attack.* It is better to prevent a heart-attack than to cause one by stressing the heart with an excessive schedule.

- **Consider Counseling** — Matters of the heart are extremely important in keeping the stress level down. We will discuss this in detail in Chapter 9.

- **Emphasize Friendship as much as Finances** — All the money in the world will not protect your heart as much as real friends. They are key to your survival and ultimate success. Cultivate friendships and create time for them — as if your life depended on it.

The recommendations are global and, of course, need to be individualized for each person's unique situation. Often overlooked, some stress reduction methods based on the wisdom of ancient medicines include:

- Yoga — the relaxing meditative kind, not the power yoga sort.

- Music — some forms of music can create an atmosphere of relaxation. Often, they imitate the relaxing impact of traditional music such as Ghandharva Veda music from India. Attentively listening to music is a way to give the mind a break.

- Playing with children — children have an innocence that does not create the normal social demand for interaction and self-consciousness. Studies in nursing homes show that the elderly who play with children have a better quality of life and better health.

- Playing with pets — animals also have a way of taking us outside of ourselves in a way that can decrease stress.

All of these recommendations can help to decrease stress. But, none is as important as the impact of meditation. Meditation addresses a major contributor to heart disease that is often overlooked. Stress is a potent killer —one that needs to be addressed directly by anyone seriously committed to maintaining a healthy heart. If we shifted even one-half of the money we currently spend on cholesterol-related efforts to stress reduction, we would make a huge impact on the health of the nation. The benefits of stress reduction would extend far beyond reducing cardiovascular disease.

* 7 *
FOOD FOR THE HEART

Confusion Abounds

Arguably, in no other facet of American culture is there as much confusion as there is about food. New diet programs sprout up daily. Yet the rate of obesity in the population continues to spiral ever higher. Advocates for a "low-fat, low-cholesterol diet" compete with the proponents of "low-carbohydrate, high-protein" regimens. The medical profession assumes that a high-protein, high-fat diet will cause cholesterol levels to spin out of control and warns the public against such an approach. Later, they observe that cholesterol levels do not necessarily rise with high-protein diets. Who's opinion can we trust?

For each recommendation that is made, a new finding negates it. For example, in the midst of the fat-free campaign spurned by the fear of cholesterol, margarine was touted to be the heart-healthy alternative to butter. But soon after, margarine was found to contain molecules (trans-fatty acids) that the body could not break down or process easily. No wonder there is confusion in the general populace about what makes a healthy diet. It is no surprise that people gravitate toward fad diets.

The standard American diet — meat-based, highly processed, and rich in fat — has little historic foundation. It is not based on any particular cultural tradition. In the history of humankind, never has this quantity and quality of the food been so readily available. The movie *Super Size Me* speaks to this issue. Frankly, some consider the American diet a huge experiment that future generations will hopefully not judge too harshly. At best, future generations may shake their heads and say: "What were our ancestors thinking?"

The changing landscape of medical nutrition puts everyone on a shaky foundation. The standard recommendations come in the form of more and more restrictions — a list of what cannot be eaten. One seldom hears a physician say that it is important to derive enjoyment, as well as nourishment, from our food. Diet has become associated with hard work, discipline, and punitive restrictions. This approach would not be so bad if the recommendations did not keep shifting. First, oils are bad; then, fish oils are good. First, cholesterol is bad; then, *some* cholesterol is good. First, it is one thing, then the other. It is no wonder that few are listening and that most

Americans are still trying to make sense out of what to do about their diet.

How can we start to understand the impact of food on heart health? Certainly, some of us have confidence in the diets that have existed and sustained human populations for thousands of years. Ancient medical systems have great wisdom to offer to this field, but most Americans would feel more secure with a scientific approach. Therefore, let us start with what we know for certain. Reviewing how atherosclerotic plaques form will give us a firm scientific foundation on which to base our recommendations.

The Process and the Bystander

Atherosclerosis starts with injury to the cells that line blood vessel walls. These endothelial cells are smart enough to know when an injury occurs. A series of events follow. First, they recruit blood elements called platelets to clot off any cracks in the lining of the inner wall and summon immune system cells to clean up any debris. Second, cells from the immune system (macrophages) ingest and oxidize cholesterol, creating "foam cells." Third, inflammation ensues when the immune system gets activated. Growth of the smooth muscle of the blood vessel results from this process, creating a fibrous vessel. Eventually, the blood vessel narrows impeding blood flow. Over time, a slab-like calcified layer forms over the injured portion of the blood vessel.

As we ascertained in Chapter 2, cholesterol does not cause atherosclerosis. It is an innocent bystander in the process. It gets recruited into atherosclerotic plaque by macrophages. One exception to this innocent bystander rule: Oxy-cholesterol. When cholesterol is oxidized, a destructive substance is created. Oxy-cholesterol is capable of damaging endothelial cells.

Clearly, the most logical approach for a diet should focus on minimizing injury to the endothelial cells, as well as avoiding the inflammatory process. Given our knowledge of the process of atherosclerosis, let us logically deduce a common-sense approach to a heart-saving diet.

Out of the Deep Fry into the Fire

How do we avoid oxy-cholesterol? First of all, realize since cholesterol is not manufactured by plants, it can only be found in animal products — meat, milk, butter, eggs. Oxy-cholesterol is created when cholesterol is exposed to temperatures of 250-260 degrees Fahrenheit or higher. If we want to keep our arteries healthy, then the implication is clear: Cooking methods are as important as what we choose to eat.

Deep frying is disastrous because it oxidizes any cholesterol that might be present in food. In fact, most cooking methods for meat are problematic. This explains one of the reasons why a meat-based diet is a setup for unhealthy arteries.

Oxy-cholesterol is created when meats are cooked. Heating cholesterol above 260 degrees creates oxy-cholesterol. Therefore, cooking meat results in oxy-cholesterol unless the animal tissues are parboiled. Boiling meat in a broth will not create as many problems as frying.

Oxy-cholesterol can be "hidden" in many of our processed foods. It appears in our baked goods in the form of powdered eggs and milk, and butter. Typically people will give up natural sources of fat, such as butter and milk, when they embark on improving their health by lowering cholesterol. But, unbeknownst to them, they ingest large quantities of oxy-cholesterol and other unnatural products. These most often sneak into our diet in the form of low-fat cookies, low-fat desserts, and low-fat crackers that have been made with powdered milk, powdered eggs, and refined flours devoid of important vitamins. The oxy-cholesterol and the lack of important B vitamins actually make the "low-fat" foods more damaging to the arteries than the unadulterated high-fat foods. To make matters worse, partially hydrogenated oils are used as substitutes for natural oils. This creates another wave of assault on the blood vessels (see section below on oils).

What To Do

Avoiding deep frying and high temperature cooking is one way of preventing the creation of oxy-cholesterol. Do not fry things in butter or clarified butter (ghee) either. Fried foods are prohibited, particularly with the dish contains any meat or butter.

Does that mean that meat is beneficial, as long as it is par-boiled? Not exactly. There are several other problems with meat. One of the main problems has to do with homocysteine. Recall from Chapter 3 that homocysteine has a potent damaging effect on endothelial cells.

Two Oxidized Burgers and Fries, Please!

Oxidation occurs rapidly when oils get old or when they are exposed to high temperatures in the cooking process. When that burger is fried, it gets oxidized. This process generates a potent source of free radicals that can cause inflammation. The cholesterol in the burger also gets damaged and becomes plaque-producing (atherogenic).

When you ingest the burger and fries, you are taking in oxy-cholesterol that has the potential to damage arteries. The fries act like a sponge, absorbing the free radicals and trans-fatty acids in the cooking oil and carrying them into your body. You also take in a good dose of methionine in the meat which gets converted to toxic homocysteine. Cooking at high temperature creates other toxic compounds, as well, such as acrylamide (a cancer-causing substance).

A diet high in vegetables provides the body with a great natural source of antioxidants. Vegetarians are also not getting as much exposure to oxidized cholesterol. Additionally, a low-animal-protein diet results in lower homocysteine levels in the blood.

The Homocysteine Story

Kilmer McCully, M.D., is considered the father of the homocysteine theory of heart disease. An observant scientist with training in biochemistry, genetics, and pathology, he became curious about a genetic disease called homocystinuria. As early as 1968, he posited that homocysteine was the culprit in the creation of damage to blood vessel walls.

Protein is composed of amino acids. One of these amino acids is methionine. It is an essential amino acid, which means it must be ingested in the food. Methionine is used to create the physical structure of the body, in other words, muscle mass. The body can take methionine and convert it to another essential amino acid called cysteine. Likewise, cysteine can be converted to methionine. However, these biochemical conversions are not straightforward. An intermediary product has to be produced first. Homocysteine is the intermediary product in the *interconversion* between methionine and cysteine.

Some people have a genetic defect that causes the normal conversion process to go haywire. Consequently, they produce large amounts of homocysteine in the blood and in the urine. Normally, homocysteine is only present in trace amounts in the blood.

A Child with Severe Atherosclerosis

At a genetics conference, Dr. McCully heard about a 9-year-old girl with homocystinuria. In describing the medical history of the family, it was explained that her uncle died at the age of 8 due to a stroke. At autopsy, they found this boy's arteries to be clogged with atherosclerosis, as if he were elderly. That case had been published in the *New England Journal of Medicine* in 1933 and had referenced the hospital where the study of the case had been undertaken — Massachusetts General Hospital, the place where McCully was employed. He went to the archives and confirmed from microscopic slides and small preserved fragments of the organs that the boy did indeed have arteriosclerosis.

What McCully realized in 1968 was that the plaques showed no evidence of cholesterol or fat deposits. He reasoned that homocysteine had caused the damage to the artery wall, but that there had not been enough time for the fat and cholesterol deposits to develop. He later confirmed the same findings in another case of elevated homocysteine in a child. This second case served as proof of his theory that the amino acid homocysteine caused atherosclerosis by directly damaging the cells and tissues of the arteries. But there is more to the story.

As previously stated, the interconversion of methionine to homocysteine to cysteine and back again does not take place in a vacuum. Biochemical processes often require enzymes or cofactors to facilitate the conversion. The cofactors required to convert the toxic substance (homocysteine) to one of its nontoxic cousins (methionine or cysteine) are the following: vitamins B6, B12, and folic acid. In fact, the genetic defect in the second child McCully studied had a problem with the function of B12.

Folic Acid and B Vitamins

In formulating his theory, McCully recalled the work of pathologist James Rhinehard who had done several experiments on monkeys. Rhinehard demonstrated that restricting vitamin B6 in the diet resulted in arteriosclerosis in these animals. McCully also found other studies in experiments with rats where vitamins B12 and folic acid were restricted and again the results showed unequivocally that arteriosclerosis was the result.

How had science missed this important connection? Arteriosclerosis and atherosclerosis were characterized by the Russian pathologist Rudolph Virchow in the 19th century. He noticed the influx of immune cells and proposed the theory that atherosclerosis was the result of some infection, as there were obvious signs of inflammation present. His theory of infection and inflammation is particularly relevant to what we now understand is the role of inflammatory markers such as C-reactive protein (CRP) in predicting artery disease.

As we discussed in Chapter 3, Dr. Harry Newburgh did experiments in the 1920s that proved a direct relationship between increasing amounts of dietary protein and increasing atherosclerosis. The more protein he fed his rabbits, the faster they developed artery disease. However, when he was unable to prove that feeding individual amino acids to the rabbits caused atherosclerosis, his theory was abandoned. Unfortunately, two amino acids had not yet been discovered at the time — methionine and homocysteine. Consequently, the cholesterol myth prevailed.

145

It was in 1969 that McCully formally proposed his homocysteine theory of heart disease. Although he was almost ostracized by the medical community, he fortunately persisted, and today research studies have proven him correct. An elevated homocysteine level is a strong risk factor for heart disease.

What is the relationship between cholesterol and homocysteine? The same lipoprotein particle that transports cholesterol throughout the body is also a carrier of homocysteine. This may explain why there is a relationship (even though weak) between markedly elevated cholesterol levels and arteriosclerosis.

> *Animal protein is high in methionine, the precursor of artery-damaging homocysteine.*

How do we avoid this artery-damaging substance? Two strategies are important. The first is to lower the intake of animal proteins that are high in methionine. The second is to avoid processed foods that are devoid of the vitamins B6, B12, and folic acid (and eat your vegetables!).

What sources of protein are high in methionine? Animal protein. Given that meat is a source of high methionine, then what can we advise about high-protein, low-carb diets? It is best to avoid them.

Because the medical community has focused so much attention on the cholesterol myth, proponents of the low-carbohydrate, high-protein diet may seem to have been vindicated. Atkins stated that a high-protein, low-carb diet would *not* significantly raise cholesterol levels. The current evidence says that he was right. However, this thinking adheres to the myth that cholesterol is the problem to begin with. If we understand that oxy-cholesterol and homocysteine are the real instigators of atherosclerosis, then we must take a more scientific view.

Low-carb, High-protein Diet

What happens to the normal function of the cells that create the inner lining of arteries (endothelium) as a result of a low-carbohydrate diet? To answer this question, the Fleming Heart and Health Institute and the Camelot Foundation in Omaha, Nebraska, looked at the effect of a high-protein diet on the blood vessels of the heart.

Twenty-six people were studied using electronic imaging techniques and ultrasound scan of the heart and other blood studies. Sixteen of the 26 had a standard low-fat diet. Ten ate a high-protein, low-carbohydrate diet.

Bad News

After one year patients in the high-protein group showed a worsening of their condition and the markers for artery disease. Specifically, C-reactive protein (CRP) increased 61 percent. Fibrinogen, a substance involved in the clotting process, increased 14 percent. Lipoprotein (a), a type of lipoprotein associated with artery disease, increased *106 percent!* The progression of coronary artery disease was documented in each of the vascular territories under study. In the high-protein group there was an overall progression of 39.7 percent.[1] On the other hand, patients in the low-fat diet group had a *regression* in the extent and severity of their disease as well as improvement in heart muscle function.

> *High-protein diets may cause progression of coronary artery disease.*

The results showed that high-protein diets may precipitate progression of coronary artery disease by increasing inflammation, clot formation, and the deposition of fat on blood vessel walls. Like the rabbits on a high-protein diet, humans also risk damage to their arteries by taking a high-protein, low-carbohydrate diet. These diets are a large experiment that are proving to be extremely dangerous.

Eating Meat may be Hazardous to the Heart

Two harmful substances are present in meat: oxy-cholesterol and high methionine levels. Methionine can be converted to the injurious homocysteine molecule. One might conclude, then, that a vegetarian diet would be superior in terms of artery health. In fact, in study after study, vegetarians are clearly found to have better cardiovascular health.

McCully states in his book, *The Heart Revolution*, that vegetarians are generally protected from atherosclerosis. He further explains: "Vegetable proteins derived from grains, beans, peas, and other vegetables contain less methionine than protein derived from meat, fish, and dairy products, so less homocysteine is produced in the body. In addition, a vegetarian diet usually contains large amounts of B vitamins, so homocysteine levels are minimized by the vitamins."[2] And again, later in the book, he writes, "The advantage for vegetarians is that plant proteins supply a lower level of methionine than animal products, and so they're at a lower risk of arteriosclerosis and heart disease to begin with. A vegetarian diet also contains more folic acid, vitamin B6, minerals, fiber, and phytochemicals, and so homocysteine is generally kept quite low."[3]

Unfortunately, McCully does not outright advocate eliminating animal protein. Instead he emphasizes getting enough vitamins from whole grains and unprocessed foods to try to handle the high methionine load from this animal protein. Perhaps this is because McCully believes that plant protein is inferior to animal protein.

In her book, *Diet for a Small Planet*, Frances Moore-Lappe popularized the idea that vegetable protein is inferior to animal protein because it does not contain the right proportion of essential amino acids. However, in a later version of her classic book, she revised her position. She showed that a vegetarian has to virtually starve or subsist on a single grain or bean in order to become deficient in essential amino acids.

The Health-Food Junkies Were Right

Whether you look at the dietary recommendations that McCully makes in his book or the dietary guidelines of the American Cancer Society, you begin to get the picture. Perhaps the "health food" advocates of the late '60s and early '70s were not just another protest group "fighting the establishment." They might have actually been onto something.

McCully explains that a major cause of heart disease has been the refining and overprocessing of food. He advocates whole foods, whole grains, and foods that are freshly prepared. He points out that refining whole wheat into white flour results in a loss of 79 percent of the folic acid and 82 percent of the B6 in the food. If you eat canned instead of fresh vegetables, you lose 57 percent of the vitamin B6 and between 57 and 84 percent of the folic acid.[4] Even freezing destroys some of the vitamin content of vegetables. He even suggests grinding your own flour to get the maximal amount of vitamins. Processed foods are not just full of preservatives and artificial flavoring; they are devoid of essential vitamins and nutrients that are essential to heart health. It would appear that the health-food junkies were right, after all.

The Russian pathologists who first observed this connection between atherosclerosis and the wealthy class assumed that diet was at the core of the disease process. Indeed, the further we stray from a plant-based diet, the greater our risk of heart disease. Additionally, switching to a predominantly plant-based diet reduces the risk of cancer, gallbladder disease, kidney stones, and gout, just to name a few.

A simple vegetarian diet based on whole foods is best. This is not just our opinion. A recent review of the effects of exercise and diet on chronic disease had this to say about the benefits of changing to a natural, plant-based diet: "Importantly, there was no evidence of a threshold beyond which further benefits did not accrue with increasing proportions of plant-based foods in the diet."[5] In other words, you can't get too much of a good thing.

> *The further we stray from a plant-based diet, the greater our risk of heart disease.*

Revisiting the Dietary Cholesterol Connection

The shocking evidence is that the connection between dietary cholesterol and heart disease has never been proven. It has simply been assumed. Two associations set the plat form for this assumption. The first was the presence of cholesterol in atherosclerotic plaque. The second was the incidence of heart disease and stroke at a young age in patients with outrageously high cholesterol (who mostly had familial hypercholesterolemia).

Cholesterol and Atherosclerotic Plaque

With respect to the first association connecting cholesterol with atherosclerotic plaque, we have already explained that it is not cholesterol itself that is damaging to arteries. The destructive element is oxy-cholesterol. To prove this hypothesis, researchers injected cholesterol into the arteries of animals. Nothing happened. They then injected oxy-cholesterol into the arteries. The animals developed arteriosclerosis.[6] This proves that oxy-cholesterol is toxic and causes plaques (atherogenic). Dietary cholesterol does not become problematic unless it is oxidized. This happens most rapidly when it is heated to high temperatures in the presence of oxygen, as occurs with frying. Some oxidation does occur simply with the exposure of cholesterol to oxygen, but this is minimal in comparison.

Genetic Defects

The second association occurs in individuals with a genetic defect. As previously mentioned, generalizing from this population to the normal population can be fraught with error. These individuals have a defect in the receptor for LDL-cholesterol in the membrane of the liver cell. This causes the metabolism to behave abnormally and creates an abnormal predilection to the creation of atherosclerosis. For these individuals, the liver cells metabolize cholesterol differently. Thus, special considerations are needed. For the rest of us, the treatment should be to avoid oxy-cholesterol and methionine. The prescribed diet is this: mostly vegetarian, based on whole grains and unprocessed foods.

Oils, Fats, and other Nonsense

Since the dietary cholesterol theory of heart disease was first introduced, the standard recommendations from the medical community have varied tremendously. Nowhere has this been greater than in the discussion of dietary fat. The campaign against butter and saturated fats made the entire U.S. move toward margarine and partially hydrogenated polyunsaturated oils. The Lyon Diet-Heart Study was one justification for this move.

Researchers from Lyon, France, proposed a "Mediterranean diet" as a heart-healthy diet. They recommended margarine made from rapeseed oil. The thinking was that the high levels of alpha-linolenic acid would be protective against heart disease.[7] The result of this diet was a lowering in the death rate from heart disease. But what is not clear from the study is which component made the greatest contribution. Was it the margarine? Was it the increase in fish consumption? The decrease in meat consumption was not clearly quantified and, obviously from the discussion above, could have played a role. The results, however, were interpreted as support for utilizing margarine, a conclusion that was disastrous.

The body lacks the ability to efficiently break down the trans-oils from which many margarines are made. These trans-oils get stored away, clogging up the body and creating fat stores that are essentially unusable. When these oils get incorporated into cells, the cells cannot function properly. In an analysis from the Nurses' Health Study, for each increase of 2 percent of energy from trans-oils, the relative risk of coronary artery

Gumming Up the Works

Margarine is made from polyunsaturated oils like corn, soybean, and sunflower oils. In order to get these oils to solidify, they need to be heated to 300–400 degrees, mixed with nickel powder, and the entire mixture is gassed with hydrogen. This process reconfigures the hydrogen atoms around the carbon double-bonds. Most oils are long chains of carbon with hydrogen atoms surrounding them. When all the carbon atoms are connected by just one single bond, then the oil is said to be saturated. When a double-bond is formed, then two hydrogen atoms are missing. This is considered a monounsaturated oil. When more than one double-bond is formed, it is considered a polyunsaturated oil. These oils do not naturally harden at room temperature. Therefore, some processing is required to make them solidify. This processing creates a problem for the body.

The Configurations

Normally, there are two hydrogen atoms per carbon (except at the ends of the carbon chains). When a double bond is formed between carbon atoms, then there is only room for one hydrogen atom on each of the carbons that form the double bond. This situation creates two possible configurations, one with the hydrogen atoms on the same side (called the *cis* configuration) or one with the atoms opposite one another (called the *trans* configuration). The interesting thing is that when the hydrogen atoms are in the trans position, the oil tends to harden, as occurs in margarines. The natural cis position does not solidify. The body lacks the ability to efficiently break down trans-oils. Margarine and trans-oils simply "gum up the works."

disease increased by 93 percent.[8] Surprisingly, total fat intake itself was not related to the risk of coronary disease.

Trans-oils have become ubiquitous. They are in baked goods, cookies, cakes, and deep-fried foods. They are disguised under the name "partially hydrogenated oils." Again, a simple diet without processed foods is much safer. Considering the average American gets more than 30 percent of calories (food energy) from fats and oils, the 2 percent of calories from trans-oils in the Nurses' Health Study represents a very small amount of food. Nevertheless, if the study is correct, the consumption of these oils more than doubles your risk of heart disease. You can lower your risk by 93 percent by eliminating them from your diet. This alone far outweighs the 24 percent risk reduction you get from taking statin cholesterol drugs.

> *For each 2 percent of calories from trans-oils, the risk of coronary disease increased by 93 percent.*

Cholesterol-lowering itself pales in comparison to what can be done by simply altering the diet. What can humankind be thinking by subjecting the body to a new, artificially created substance (manufactured trans-oils) when the body has subsisted on a predominance of cis-oils for millions of years. This is a giant experiment which has turned the entire population into guinea pigs. It is no wonder the health of Americans is so poor.

The Further Cost of Free Radicals

Saturated fats, those without any double bonds, include butter, lard, and oils like coconut oil. These were "replaced" by margarines and "partially hydrogenated oils." Saturated fats became the bad guys because they supposedly increased that alleged "toxic" substance, cholesterol.

Saturated Oils

It turns out that saturated oils may not be the bad guys after all. Let us compare them to some of the unsaturated oils. Monounsaturated oils are oils like olive oil and canola oil. Polyunsaturated oils include safflower, sunflower, and corn oils.

The saturated oils have no carbon-carbon double bonds whereas the polyunsaturated oils do. This double bond gives the polyunsaturated oils the capability of reacting with neighboring molecules. The double bond is highly reactive and can "steal electrons" from neighboring molecules. In the process, these highly charged bonds create "free radicals." Recall from Chapter 3 that free radicals are destructive actors that can damage endothelial cells and start the whole process of atherosclerosis. This tendency for polyunsaturated oils to create free radicals may help explain why animal studies have shown these oils to be carcinogenic.[9] When these oils are kept at high temperature for hours (as in a deep fryer in a fast-food restaurant), their ability to produce cancer in animals increases.[10]

Polyunsaturated oils can produce destruction in two ways. The free radicals they create can cause damage to the endothelial cells. Additionally, the oils themselves can also come into contact with the body's own cholesterol (or other cholesterol in the diet) and create oxy-cholesterol. Given the current craze about avoiding saturated fats, most people will be surprised to know that the Framingham Study actually showed a *decrease* in the risk of stroke with saturated fats and monounsaturated oils, whereas increased intake of polyunsaturated fats did nothing to decrease the risk of stroke.[11]

A study of dietary fats in postmenopausal women concluded that polyunsaturated fats may actually be worse than saturated fats. The coronary arteries from 235 women with known heart disease were examined via a sophisticated electronic imaging technique (quantitative coronary angiography) at the beginning of the study and then again 3.1 years later. The mean total fat intake was 25 percent (plus or minus 6 percent) of all calories taken. Researchers found that higher saturated fat intake was associated with less narrowing of the artery.[12] This trend was especially strong in those who took lower amounts of monounsaturated fat and higher carbohydrates.

Dietary intake of polyunsaturated fats was associated with progression of atherosclerosis when it was used to replace other fats in the diet; but, interestingly enough, not when it was used to replace calories from protein or from carbohydrate. Perhaps, the advantages and benefits of less homocysteine from protein were offset by the increase in free radicals from polyunsaturated fats, making the whole thing a wash.

The authors concluded that, in postmenopausal women with relatively low fat intake, higher saturated fat intake was associated with less progression of coronary artery disease.

These results buttress research done in India where large quantities of ghee (clarified butter) are sometimes incorporated into the diet. Researchers looked at the fat consumption of 782 rural males. Their main source of fat was ghee and mustard/rapeseed oil. Analysis of the diets of these men showed that the group that consumed more ghee had 23 percent less chance of developing coronary artery disease.[13]

> *Olive oil is the best monounsaturated oil.*

Olive oil is the best monounsaturated oil. It does not seem wise to take a chemically-detoxified, genetically-engineered rapeseed oil like canola oil. Stick with olive oil or ghee (just don't fry it). When you buy olive oil, be sure to get virgin, cold-pressed, *unrefined* oil. Otherwise, it may be processed, just like most of the commercially available canola oil.

Fishy Business

Oils such as safflower, sunflower, peanut, and corn oil are polyunsaturated oils that have the unsaturated double bond at the sixth carbon. They are said to belong to the "omega-6" family of polyunsaturated oils. While they tend to lower serum cholesterol levels slightly, animal studies have shown

Would You Give This Oil To Your Dog?

Take a plant by the name of rapeseed. Now, if you wanted to extract an oil from it for human consumption, you would be out of luck. Unfortunately, it contains high levels or erucic acid. Erucic acid has been thought to create fatty hearts as well as thyroid and adrenal degeneration in rats. So, in order to reduce the level of erucic acid from the normal 5 percent or higher to 1 percent, you have to breed out the plant. Thus far, you might actually have an edible oil.

But, how do you get large quantities of the oil out of the plant? Following the typical procedure used by oil producers, you cook the seeds at about 248 degrees. This process creates cracks in the seeds and the resultant exposure to air creates some rancidity; but, the yield is much greater (you can take care of the rancidity later). Next, you take the cooked seeds and mechanically press them under extremely high pressures. This creates its own heat, usually up to 195 degrees Fahrenheit, and further oxidizes the oil. If you want "unrefined" oil, you stop here.

Usually 9–18 percent of the oil is still in the pressed seed meal that is left over after mechanical compression. To extract that, you use a solvent. If you are like a lot of oil producers, you use hexane or heptane as a solvent (yes, that is right, gasoline!). Then you have to boil off the solvent, once again heating the oil and creating more rancidity. Now in order to get usable oil, you need to degum it, refine it, bleach it, and deodorize it. Degumming can be done by heating It to 140 degrees with water and phosphoric acid. Refining occurs when the oil is mixed with an extremely corrosive base, such as sodium hydroxide (yes, that is right, it is the same as what is in Drano!). The mixture is agitated and then allowed to separate. Bleaching requires heating it to 230 degrees for 15 to 30 minutes and passing it through acid–treated activated clays or fuller's earth. This creates some toxic peroxides and conjugated fatty acids. Deodorizing is done under steam distillation at 464–518 degrees for 30–60 minutes.

This causes some of the fatty acids in the oil to transform to trans-fatty acids and also creates changes in the oil that are considered by some to be capable of damaging genes (mutagenic). Deodorization removes the peroxides produced during refining and bleaching.

You now have an oil that you can sell. But first, you must give it a name that sounds healthy ... say, something that rhymes with "granola." Yes, this is how canola oil is made. Canola is Canadian rapeseed oil. To make matters worse, a genetically-engineered rapeseed plant has been developed that is being used in Canada.

Now if that doesn't make you think twice about the "health benefits" of canola oil, consider this. This modified rapeseed oil still contains some erucic acid. It has never before in the history of humankind been used for widespread consumption, as it is a modified, specially bred plant. It is not the same plant that is used in Asia to create rapeseed oil. It represents in essence a giant experiment with the public as guinea pigs. Would you feed it to your dog?

Mustard/rapeseed oil is not usually well-recognized by Americans. This is a result of the clever marketing undertaken by food producers. Canola oil is more well-recognized. The name "canola" was created to avoid the more distasteful word "rapeseed." Canola oil is a monounsaturated oil and therefore theoretically less toxic than polyunsaturated oils. But, canola oil poses great health hazards unless it is cold-pressed, unrefined. The entire extraction process can create more free radicals. Avoid the experiment and do not consume canola oil.

that a high intake of these oils is potentially cancer-producing.[14,15] Heating these oils makes them become rancid quickly. Many commercially available oils are, in fact, deodorized to mask their rancidity.

Fish oils have been researched extensively. They have the main unsaturated bond at the third carbon. They are known, therefore, as "omega-3 oils." Omega-3 oils lower levels of blood homocysteine. They also tend to reduce the number of free radicals produced. This is important because oxidative stress creates free radicals. Taking too much omega-6 oils in the diet can upset the benefit of taking omega-3 oils. The ratio is important as a high omega-6/omega 3 ratio creates inflammation in the body.

Oils are inherently inflammatory in nature. There are four exceptions to this rule: ghee (clarified butter), coconut, olive, and fish oils. Recall that inflammation is what keeps the process of atherosclerosis in motion.

Fire in the Vessels

Damage to the artery wall is promoted by homocysteine and oxy-cholesterol. But that is only the first part of the story. For the injury to cause thickening (scleroses) of the arteries, the immune system must get involved. The result is inflammation. This is why those with signs of inflammation, such as elevated C-reactive protein (CRP), are at greater risk for heart attack. What does food have to do with the immune system?

From the standard medical standpoint, the connection between food and inflammation has remained relatively ignored. However, the recent interest in CRP and the recognition of the "metabolic syndrome" has provided a definite connection between these two. The metabolic syndrome is a collection of metabolic derangements that occur in the face of insulin resistance.

Weight Concerns

In some individuals, the body responds to excess weight with changes in how it handles blood sugar. In order for cells to utilize blood sugar for energy, they require insulin to "turn the key." Insulin unlocks the doors into the cell that allow for sugar to be utilized. With chronic overweight, insulin resistance is created. The cells act as if they were "full" and do not need more blood sugar and resist incorporating it into their cells. The pancreas is forced to produce higher and higher levels of insulin to get blood sugar into the cells. When it can no longer keep up, blood sugar levels rise resulting in diabetes.

Understand that all carbohydrates (grains, starch, breads) break down into simple sugar molecules called glucose. When carbohydrates are not taken in the diet, the liver creates blood sugar from stores of glycogen. It can actually create sugar from fat or protein. The brain must have a constant supply of blood sugar in order to function properly. Consequently, the body is designed to use many different sources of food by converting these foods into sugar.

The Metabolic Syndrome

High levels of insulin and insulin resistance is only one aspect of a whole set of problems that occur as a result of excess weight. This set of problems is called the metabolic syndrome. Other aspects of the syndrome include increased levels of circulating cholesterol, triglycerides, lipoproteins, and also a tendency toward increased blood pressure. Individuals with the metabolic syndrome are at high risk for heart disease. Increased levels of insulin stimulate smooth muscle proliferation. This means that the smooth muscle in the arteries in areas of inflammation enlarge and block off more of the artery.

The increased levels of insulin and blood sugar are also associated with cytokines being released by fat cells. Cytokines are chemical messengers that stimulate the immune system. The metabolic syndrome results in vascular endothelial dysfunction, an abnormal lipid profile, hypertension, and vascular inflammation. All of these factors promote the development of atherosclerotic disease.[16,17,18]

The metabolic syndrome is sometimes seen in individuals who have a "normal" weight, but have abdominal obesity. In fact, part of the formal definition of the metabolic syndrome is a waist circumference greater than 40 inches in men and greater than 35 inches in women. Another definition includes a waist to hip ratio greater than 0.90.

The metabolic syndrome has been recognized as a pro-inflammatory and prothrombotic (blood clot forming) state. It is associated with elevated levels of C-reactive protein, interleukin-6 (a cytokine that stimulates the immune system), and plasminogen activator inhibitor-1 (another clotting-related factor).[19,20] All these things contribute to atherosclerosis, and those with the metabolic syndrome are at high risk for artery disease.[21,22]

How much does the metabolic syndrome increase the risk of heart disease? A great deal. Here are a few of the studies that have examined the increase in risk due to this syndrome:

- In the Scotland trial (WOSCOPS), individuals with the metabolic syndrome increased their risk of cardiovascular disease by 1.8. Among men, if they had four or five features of the formal definition of metabolic syndrome (see below), their risk increased 3.7 fold when compared to men with no features of the syndrome.[23]

- Among 1,200 men in Finland followed for 11 years, those with the metabolic syndrome at baseline had a 4.2-fold increased relative risk of coronary heart disease death and a 2.0-fold increased relative risk of all-cause mortality compared with men without the syndrome.[24]

- Among subjects in the placebo arms of the secondary prevention 4S trial and the primary prevention AFCAPS/TexCAPS trial, the metabolic syndrome increased the relative risk of major coronary events (fatal or nonfatal MI, sudden cardiac death, or unstable angina) by about 1.5-fold.[25]

- The WISE study of 780 women showed that the metabolic syndrome was significantly associated with an overall risk increase of 2.01 (three-year risk of death or major adverse cardiovascular events).[26]

A formal definition of the metabolic syndrome has been provided to physicians in the form of the guidelines from the 2001 National Cholesterol Education Program (Adult Treatment Panel [ATP] III). Note that the formal definition of the syndrome does not include a reference to the level of "bad" (LDL) cholesterol. *In fact, the clinical definition does not even require measuring cholesterol at all.* It is based on having any three of the following:

1. Abdominal obesity defined as a waist circumference in men greater than 102 cm (40 in) and in women greater than 88 cm (35 in); or, a waist to hip ratio greater than 0.90.
2. Serum triglycerides greater than or equal to 150 mg/dL (1.7 mmol/L).
3. Serum HDL cholesterol less than 40 mg/dL (1 mmol/L) in men and less than 50 mg/dL (1.3 mmol/L) in women.
4. Blood pressure greater than or equal to 130/85 mmHg.
5. Fasting plasma glucose (FPG) greater than or equal to 110 mg/dL (6.1 mmol/L). Other authoritative panels have recently suggested this number to be lowered to greater than or equal to 100 mg/dL (5.6 mmol/L).

The different studies reporting on this syndrome recognize that cholesterol is not the culprit in causing heart disease. Other pro-inflammatory and clot-promoting metabolic processes are much more important in forming atherosclerotic plaque. These studies show that some of the inflammatory and immune system-related components that are part of the atherosclerosis process can actually be measured and detected in patients *before* the onset of heart disease.

Obviously, those with the metabolic syndrome and excess weight have a need to reduce calories and lose weight. It is a huge risk for heart disease. However, it is noteworthy that people can have normal weight and still have the metabolic syndrome. In some studies, up to 5 percent of those with normal weight showed signs of insulin resistance and the metabolic syndrome.

Why are some individuals getting insulin resistance without excessive weight? Do other things increase insulin levels? Is there something magical about the cut-off values in the definition?

The reality is that the syndrome is not an all or nothing phenomenon. It happens gradually, not like suddenly falling off a cliff. Consequently, even approaching these values for blood sugar, blood pressure, lipid levels, and weight can signal that the inflammatory process has started. When does diet become an agent of inflammation?

Not So Simple Sugars

Refined sugars are found in many foods. They have names like sucrose, dextrose, corn syrup, and plain table sugar. These are otherwise considered "simple sugars." Refined sugars are the main ingredients of soft drinks. The average American consumes a half a pound of sugar each day. Simple sugars cause dramatic swings in insulin levels because they are so readily absorbed into the blood stream. They create a temporary surge in blood sugar levels that stimulates the release of insulin from the pancreas. Sometimes this release is so fast that it "overshoots" the level needed and causes the blood sugar levels to drop dramatically. When the blood sugar goes too low, it creates the "crash" and fatigue that comes after the "sugar high."

High insulin levels cause atherosclerosis by promoting the growth of smooth muscle cells in the arteries. This whole metabolic swing creates a situation that fosters inflammation. In fact, middle-aged women with normal weight who consume large quantities of refined carbohydrates have been found to have elevated C-reactive protein levels.[27] Additionally, eating a lot of refined sugar increases glycosylation (deposition of sugar) on red blood cells and other structures in the body as well. In order to deal with this "gumming up of the works," the body's immune system must work overtime to clean up the mess. This up-regulation of the immune system is expressed as higher levels of inflammation and elevated CRPs. Practitioners of Chinese medicine recognize this phenomenon as *Damp Heat;* those of Ayurveda, as *Toxic Ama.* But this is not the only way that refined sugars and dietary choices create inflammation and immune system involvement.

Researchers have documented the relationship between high intake of simple sugars and inflammation. Utilizing food-frequency questionnaires, Harvard researchers were able to quantify the "glycemic load" in 244 apparently healthy women. Glycemic load is a measure of the intake of rapidly digested and absorbed carbohydrates (i.e., simple sugars). A high dietary glycemic load comes from a diet high in simple sugars. A low glycemic load is associated with complex carbohydrates like those found in whole grains. After adjusting

167

for age and for other inflammatory factors like the presence of diabetes or hypertension, correlations were made between glycemic load and CRP levels. Individuals with a glycemic load in the lowest 20 percent had a mean CRP level of 1.4 mg/dL. Those with the glycemic load in the top 20 percent had a mean CRP of 3.8 mg/dL. If the weight status or body mass was taken into account, this association was even stronger.[28] This later result is very important. It shows that even in women with low or normal body weight, an increased intake of simple sugars creates more inflammation and higher CRP levels.

Simple sugars are not so simple in their metabolism. They create great swings in insulin levels and predispose to inflammation and disease. Furthermore, they take away from the consumption of complex carbohydrates — natural whole grains, that provide important B vitamins and minerals, as well as fiber.

Just the Facts — Your Dietary Guidelines

The best heart health dietary recommendations are based on what we know about the processes that damage arteries. The ABCs of the heart healthy diet are:

- **A**void free radicals — minimize the potential for free radical damage.

- **B**eware of homocysteine — minimize animal protein in the diet.

- **C**ool off the fire in your body — minimize foods that create inflammation.

Let's take each of these principles one by one and derive some concrete suggestions.

Avoid free radicals — minimize the potential for free radical damage.

Refined oils and fats are a major sources of free radicals. Cooking at high temperatures oxidizes them. To avoid this potential source of damage, the following are important:

- Do not eat any fried foods and especially avoid deep-fried foods. The oils used for deep-frying have been heated to high temperatures and this process creates potent free radicals even in vegetable oils.

- Avoid oxy-cholesterol by keeping the cooking temperature of butter or ghee at or below 212 degrees. If you sauté with these oils use a little water in the pan to prevent the temperature from going above 212 degrees.

- Avoid oxy-cholesterol by avoiding processed and baked foods. Many processed foods contain "dry milk" or "powdered eggs." The processing involved with the creation of these ingredients creates free radicals that can damage the body.

- Avoid using canola oil or any oil that is refined. The oils are processed using high temperatures. This damages the oils and they, in turn, can damage your heart. Particularly avoid salad dressings unless they are made with extra virgin, cold-extracted olive oil. It would be best to make your own fresh batch.

- Olive oil is the best oil. Second best is butter or clarified butter or ghee. (Use in small quantities only.)

- Avoid processed and baked foods that contain "partially hydrogenated" oils. These are highly processed oils that create more indigestible trans-fatty acids and are potent carriers of free radicals.

Beware of homocysteine — minimize animal protein in the diet.

Homocysteine is the intermediary product between two essential amino acids, methionine and cysteine. Animal protein contains a high concentration of methionine — the higher the protein consumption, the greater the chance of creating homocysteine. The ability of the body to convert homocysteine to its nontoxic counterparts is dependent on vitamin B6, B12, and folic acid. To minimize homocysteine and protect heart health, adhere to the following:

- Enjoy a low-protein diet. It is difficult to become protein deficient if you eat a variety of foods. There is no need to be adding protein or worrying about inadequate protein if you are consuming sufficient calories in a varied diet.

- Move toward a vegetarian diet. Vegetable sources of protein contain less methionine and therefore decrease the amount of homocysteine in the body. Moving toward a vegetarian diet means eliminating red meat and starting to explore some vegetarian meals (such as tasty ethnic foods — hummus, fettuccine Alfredo, pinto bean enchiladas). Eventually, eliminate all meat except chicken and fish. Continue exploring vegetarian alternatives for three months and then decrease the amount of chicken and fish (or eliminate chicken entirely). As much as possible, use grass-fed, organic meats.

- Avoid processed foods and favor whole grains. Whole grains contain the full amount of B vitamins and minerals. These are destroyed in the creation of white flour and refined products. The more B vitamins in your diet, the more easily homocysteine can get converted back to nontoxic amino acids.

- Consume dark leafy greens each day (for example, collards, kale, chard, Swiss chard). These are high in folic acid and also help in the conversion of homocysteine to nontoxic forms.

- Get adequate intake of vitamin C. This vitamin is an important part of the metabolic pathway that converts homocysteine to less toxic forms. When vitamin C intake is inadequate, homocysteine levels rise dangerously. Natural sources of vitamin C such as fresh citrus are much better than supplementation.

Cool off the fire in your body — minimize foods that create inflammation.

A large intake of simple sugars creates the potential for inflammation in the body. Sugars in many forms can create problems for metabolism and adversely affect health. To minimize inflammation in the body and the buildup of advanced glycosylation products (sugar deposits in the body), do the following:

- Eliminate refined sugar from the diet. Take small amounts of honey, maple syrup, or Turbinado sugar if you take any at all. Favor fruits and fruit sugar for sweeteners, as fructose is metabolized differently from sucrose (white sugar).

- Decrease the amount of calories in the diet from sugar. Eliminate soft drinks, and favor herbal teas or warm water instead.

- Increase the amount of whole grain foods in the diet. Use many types of grains besides wheat, such as barley, quinoa, amaranth, oats, millet, rice, brown basmati rice, Shushi rice, wild rice. (See *Heaven's Banquet* by Miriam Hospodar for an excellent discussion of how to cook grains and also for excellent vegetarian recipes.)

- Decrease the amount of unwholesome oils in the diet. Like throwing oil on a fire, most oils have the tendency to increase inflammation in the body. Moderate your oil intake and favor saturated oils like butter, ghee, coconut, or the monounsaturated oil (olive oil). These oils have less potential for creating free radicals.

- Get your essential fatty acids (essential oils) by eating nuts and seeds like sunflower seeds. Sprinkle fresh-ground flaxseeds in cereal or salad.

- Moderate your consumption of soy products. Soy is estrogenic, which is why it can help some women during menopause when their production of estrogen drops. As we have learned from the Women's Health Initiative, high estrogen levels predispose a woman toward more heart disease. This could result from the triggering of inflammation by estrogen. Alternatively, it could be just the tendency toward more clotting which occurs with high estrogen levels. Rarely, some women will get hepatitis or liver inflammation when put on estrogen. While the mechanism is not clearly understood, it is better to eat moderate amounts of soy and avoid its estrogenic effects.

- If you are not a vegetarian and have problems with inflammation, discuss the use of fish oils with your health-care provider.

Summary

Research indicates that a vegetarian diet can lower the risk of heart disease dramatically. A 75 percent reduction in heart disease in strict vegetarians is noted by some.[29] This reduction in risk far exceeds anything possible with drug intervention. Combining this with the other dietary changes can greatly benefit health in all aspects, not just heart health. Moving towards a vegetarian diet decreases your risk of heart disease. Knowledge of how to use oils and which oils to use, incorporating whole grains into the diet, and avoiding simple sugars, all make a tremendous impact on your overall health. This is the most heart-saving intervention you can undertake. It costs nothing. In fact, it can save you money at the grocery store. The most important interventions in preventing heart disease have nothing to do with measuring your cholesterol. By taking control of your diet, you alone can control your health, well-being, and longevity.

* 8 *
MOVEMENT

"I just don't have the discipline to exercise." So states our last patient of the day. To her, exercise must involve hard work, and she is already overworked and tired. Besides, her schedule is so packed that, even if she had the motivation, she feels she would not have the time. Exercise is yet another task for her. Her husband, who is unemployed, has been cooking all their meals. As result of his rich, meat-based meals, she has gained 25 pounds in the last year.

"You don't need more work," we explain. "You need more play in your life." Finding something that she enjoys doing that involves movement takes some time. We reviewed possible enjoyable options, including those from her childhood, as well as her adult life. Then it was easier to begin this most important process of incorporating movement into her routine.

The human body was made to move. A major portion of the brain is dedicated to movement. Without motion, the body begins to lose muscle mass and health starts to decline. Movement does not have to be exercise. It is difficult to dispel the negative associations people have with the word "exercise." During consultations, we spend extra time explaining the difference between exercise and movement; between "workouts" and "playouts." The investment of time is worth it because movement is critical to health, especially heart health. What is this belief based on?

> *The human body was made to move.*

The Science of Movement Physiology

What happens to the body when we move? In a nutshell, disease is prevented. More than 110 million Americans suffer from some chronic disease. The majority of this can be prevented. That is not just our opinion. Here is a statement from a recent medical journal summarizing the effects of exercise and diet on chronic disease:

> This review will provide evidence that when daily physical activity of one hour is performed in combination with a natural food diet, high in fiber-containing fruits, vegetables, and whole grains, and naturally low in fat, containing abundant amounts of vitamins, minerals, and phytochemicals, *the majority of chronic disease may be prevented.*[1]

The rest of the review goes on to document in great detail the effects of physical activity and diet on coronary artery disease, hypertension, diabetes, metabolic syndrome, and cancer. Note that the word "physical activity" is used. This is important, as movement does not have to be work or "exercise" in order to benefit health.

What specifically happens with physical activity that benefits health? Remember that HDL-cholesterol is thought to be "good" cholesterol and protective against heart disease. HDL-cholesterol can protect against the oxidation of LDL-cholesterol ("bad" cholesterol). Recall that cholesterol is not damaging unless it is oxidized. Roberts showed that physical activity can change the nature of HDL in people with coronary artery disease. In these people, their HDL does not protect against LDL oxidation. However, with lifestyle modification, the ability of HDL to protect against LDL oxidation improves.[2] So activity can make HDL-cholesterol a better antioxidant. It can also decrease the susceptibility of LDL-cholesterol to oxidation.

Other benefits include a decrease in C-reactive protein (CRP) levels, indicating lower levels of inflammation. Wegge and colleagues demonstrated that physical activity in conjunction with dietary intervention reduced CRP by 45 percent and decreased ICAM-1 (an immune system messenger) in post-menopausal women with risk factors for coronary artery disease.[3] Lower levels of inflammation in the body decrease the second phase of the arteriosclerosis process. In addition, the propensity toward clotting is reduced. But this is just the beginning.

Physical activity improves endothelial function, insulin resistance, immune system function, and blood pressure. Triglyercide levels tend to go down.[4] Antioxidant enzymes in the body such as superoxide dismutase and glutathione peroxidase go up.[5]

The immune system sends signals via special messenger molecules called cytokines. Some cytokines are signals associated with increased inflammation and with more promotion of the atherosclerosis process and are called atherogenic cytokines. Some cytokines decrease inflammation and protect the blood vessels from atherosclerosis. These are called "atheroprotective" cytokines. Regular physical activity was shown to decrease the atherogenic cytokines (IL-1, TNF-alpha, Interleukin-gamma) by as much as 58 percent and to increase the level of atheroprotective cytokines (IL-4, IL-10, Transforming Growth Factor-Beta-1) by as much as 36 percent.[6]

In other studies, regular physical activity was shown to improve endothelium-dependent vasodilation. This reflects the artery's ability to respond when it receives a message to dilate the vessel.[7] If the vessel cannot dilate when needed, then blood pressure goes up. High blood pressure creates a dangerous situation, which is potentially damaging for the vessel.

The improvements are so great with exercise that they surpass modern medical interventions. This was shown in a study comparing one year of exercise training with angioplasty. Angioplasty is a common procedure whereby a wire is inserted into an artery in the leg and run up to a coronary artery, one of the vessels that surround the heart. A tiny balloon on the end of the wire is used to open up the clogged artery.

The results of the study showed that the number of heart attacks (event-free survival) was less in the exercise group than in the group that received angioplasty. In fact, it was far superior. Not only were there fewer cardiac events, there was much less cost involved in the exercise training because of the reduced need for hospitalizations and the frequent need to repeat the angioplasty procedure in that group.[8]

Finally, physical activity makes maintaining optimal weight easier. It decreases the tendency toward the metabolic syndrome and helps in losing weight.

> *Exercise creates a 100 percent decrease in coronary artery disease.*

What are the implications for decreasing the risk of artery disease? The relative risk of coronary artery disease is estimated to be two-fold higher for inactive people.[9] This represents a 100 percent increase in risk as compared with those who engage in regular physical activity. Likely, this is an average estimate. Larger estimates come from studies such as the Harvard alumni study of 4,276 men. In this study the relative risk of death from coronary artery disease was approximately three-fold or 200 percent higher for inactive individuals.[10] Even 30 minutes of training with weights per week is sufficient to decrease the risk of coronary artery disease. This was shown in the Health Professionals Follow-up Study reported in 2002.[11] Compare these reductions in risk with the expense, time, and effort in taking medications for cholesterol: A 100 percent reduction with regular physical activity or a 25 percent reduction with 30 minutes per week of weight training versus a 24 percent reduction with statin drugs. Considering that the estimated 100 percent reduction may be an underestimate, the message is clear — humans were meant to move. In movement, there is health.

Movement Strategies

Exercise has become synonymous with vigorous aerobic activities, such as jogging or running. Most people are surprised to learn that many of the research studies on physical activity and the reversing of heart disease involve nothing more than walking. Walking for 45 minutes to one hour a day is all that was necessary to bring about dramatic changes in those with established coronary artery disease. For prevention, even 30 minutes of walking a day is adequate. Most people can do this without even considering it "exercise."

Physical activity just means moving. Many strategies can help to incorporate more movement into the day. Taking the stairs instead of the elevator or escalator; parking your car at the end of the parking lot, instead of right next to the building; dividing the laundry into smaller loads so that you go up and down the stairs a few extra times; riding a bike instead taking the car; walking to the end of the plant or the office instead of phoning — these are strategies that can serve to enhance your physical well-being without the effort of "working out."

If allotting time for physical activity is an issue, then we recommend that you do it first thing in the day. That way, regardless of what happens during the day, you have already performed this essential task. You have made health the first priority of your day. What is crucial in this approach is to recognize that movement does not have to be work. Here is a list of so-called "exercise" methods that are not in the category of a "workout":

- Rhythmically moving around in the comfort of your living space
- Ballroom dancing
- Gardening
- Housecleaning (sweeping, scrubbing floors, etc.)
- Skating
- Tai chi
- Yoga
- Playing frisbee
- Skipping
- Jumping rope
- Dancing
- Raking leaves
- Shoveling snow

- Biking

- Handball, squash, tennis

- Walking the dog

Many ordinary tasks of daily living can be undertaken as a way of enhancing physical activity. Instead of using a gasoline-powered lawnmower, use an old-fashioned push-mower. If this approach does not suit you, then find something that is fun to do. For many dancing is a joy, not work. Dancing is a wonderful way to get exercise and to enjoy moving.

Movement is a fun part of human existence. Find a way to enjoy playing again. Consider some of the old games you played as a child (playing in the water, jumping rope) or things that might be attractive to you as an adult, such as yoga or tai chi. Finally, for those who enjoy more vigorous training, be careful to start a new training program in a gradual, measured way. Check with your physician or health-care provider before starting.

> *The axiom "no pain, no gain" is simply false.*

The axiom "no pain, no gain" is *not* correct. When pain is induced, stress is created. As we pointed out in earlier chapters, stress creates heart disease. Training can involve anything from swimming to biking to jogging. Some guidelines that come from alternative and ancient medical systems, such as Ayurvedic medicine, may help if you want to train:

- Measure your resting heart rate first thing in the morning. If it goes up by five beats per minute, you have overdone the workout the day before. Consequently, you should skip a day of training.

- Your maximal heart rate during exercise should not exceed 130 beats per minute.

- Breathe through your nose while exercising. If you are working so hard that you have to breathe through your mouth, then you are overdoing it.

- Train in the morning — working out at night elevates the core body temperature at a time when it naturally declining to prepare the body for sleep. Working out at night can be a prescription for sleep disturbance. Working out at lunchtime will create digestion problems. Morning is the best time with late afternoon being second-best.

Do whatever it takes to enjoy moving — do it! You will reap tremendous benefits. Schedule this as you would any important meeting. Truth be told: It is the most important meeting of the day.

* 9 *
HEART MATTERS

The Heart as a Metaphor

The heart is a muscular pump with attached tubing, technically speaking. It functions to move blood to the rest of the body with the use of electrical impulses and physical force. In simple terms, then, is there any difference between the electric water pump in your house and the heart you house in your body?

Perhaps it is the sages and the poets, not the anatomists, who have best understood the function of the heart. The "heart" is the source of a person's feelings and emotions. The heart serves as a metaphor for the seat of human emotion. Our everyday language is speckled with idioms reflecting this point.

Whether the generator of emotion or a physical pump, scientific evidence asserts that the metaphorical heart influences the state of the physical pump. It might be, therefore, more than a figure of speech to say that a person died of a "broken heart."

> *Mounting scientific evidence demonstrates that emotions affect the state of the muscular pump.*

The following section explores the effects of psychological and social factors on the health of the physical heart. In general, review of available literature revealed three major themes. Each of these themes may be, in turn, considered a "risk factor" in determining the likelihood of heart disease. The three themes are as follows:

1) Lack of social connectedness;
2) Sense of loss, depression and hopelessness; and
3) Mental and emotional stress leading to anger and anxiety.

The Health-Damaging Consequences of Negative Emotions

Risk Factor #1: Loneliness

It has been said that humans were not meant to be alone nor without someone who understands them. Social connections provide individuals with a sense of belonging whereby members form a network of mutual responsibility. In this context, the individual perceives being cared for, loved, and esteemed. Social connectedness subsequently yields social support.

Social support may take the form of emotional, informational, or instrumental support. Emotional support involves the verbal and nonverbal communication of being cared for, valued, loved, and needed. Informational support takes the form of access to information, advice, appraisal, and guidance from others. Instrumental support involves access to material and physical assistance (i.e., money, help with tasks, functional aid).[1]

Social connectedness may occur in many ways and can involve many different sources. It occurs with our selves, a significant other, relatives, a community of friends, or members of other species (i.e., animals/pets). A deep source of connection may be with a spiritual force or simply, but powerfully, with our spiritual Self through meditation and prayer.

Can Your Community Save Your Mortal Heart?

The population of Roseto, Pennsylvania, was studied extensively for 50.[2] This community was found to have a strikingly low mortality rate from heart disease, especially when compared to two immediately adjacent towns (Bangor and Nazareth). Of note, the medically recognized risk factors for heart disease were equally prevalent in all three. The social structure of this community was determined to afford its members a protective factor against heart disease.

Unlike its neighbors, the population in Roseto benefited from a high level of ethnic and social homogeneity, close family ties, and cohesive community relationships during the first 30 years of the study. Roseto was settled by immigrants from a town in southern Italy in 1882. Later, in the late 1960s and early '70s, Roseto shifted away from three-generation households with strong commitment to religion, relationships, and traditional values. With this shift came a substantial increase in death and disease. The incidence of heart disease paralleled the growth of community fragmentation and social isolation.[3]

In another powerful case, researchers studied 12,000 Japanese individuals.[4] This heart disease study researched the effect of living in Japan versus Honolulu or San Francisco. Data revealed that the incidence of heart disease was related to two factors: (1) proximity to the homeland and (2) the degree to which individuals retained a traditional Japanese culture. Prevalence of heart disease was less in Japanese individuals living in Japan even though there is a higher incidence of smoking there. The individuals who retained less of their traditional culture, including looser social networks, family ties, and community, had a *three- to five-fold* increase in heart disease.[5]

Can Social Ties Keep Your Heart Alive?

Four extensive studies explored the relationship between social connection and survival. All the studies found that individuals who were either classified or perceived themselves to be isolated were at higher risk of death.

The combination of social isolation and a high degree of life stress imparted *four* times the risk of death. This was the case even when controlling for other prognostic factors. The 2,300 male heart-attack survivors were also on medication (beta-blockers) to control hypertension. This fact revealed yet another interesting association. Social isolation and stress had a more profound influence on total deaths and sudden cardiac deaths than the use of heart medication.[6]

Another study involved 13,000 people in Finland with traditional cardiovascular risk factors. Over a period of five to nine years, those men who were socially isolated suffered an increased risk of death. They were *two to three* times at higher risk of death than those men who reported the highest sense of social connection and community.[7]

Group affiliation predicted the likelihood of mortality in a study of 2,000 men from Evan County, Georgia. Results revealed that marriage, contact with extended family and friends, and church membership was associated with decreased mortality. This association was demonstrated after 11 to 13 years of follow-up study and even after adjusting for confounding factors. Moreover, loss of social connections was predictive of increased risk of death due to heart disease.[8]

Individuals who lacked regular participation in organized social groups had a four-fold increased risk of dying six months after surgery. Likewise, those who reported not drawing strength and comfort from their religion or spiritual faith were three times more likely to die. These two factors had an independent and additive effect, increasing risk of death by *seven* times.[9]

Can Pouring Love into Your Heart Keep Your Coronary Arteries Open?

Two studies evaluated the effect of being loved and supported on the blockage of the arteries of the heart. Both found that availability of deep emotional relationships and the perception of being loved by someone predicted the severity of disease. This effect was independent of diet, smoking, hypertension, exercise, cholesterol levels, family history of heart disease, or other standard risk factors.[10,11]

Can Baring Your Heart to Someone Keep You Alive?

Emotional intimacy is lifesaving. This is the take-home message of a study involving 1,400 men and women who were diagnosed with at least one severely blocked coronary artery.

Five years after this initial finding, 50 percent of those who were unmarried and without a confidant died. Also, they were *three* times more likely to die than their married counterparts.[12]

Can a Wife's Show of Love Lessen Heartache?

Ten thousand married men who were at-risk of developing heart disease were evaluated based on the standard risk factors. Of the individuals who developed angina in the next five years, the stronger predictor of their degree of chest pain was the answer to one question in their initial evaluation: "Does your wife show you her love?" Those who answered in the affirmative had significantly less chest pain. Demonstration of love by the spouse appeared to have a buffering effect against harmful risk factors such as cholesterol, blood pressure, anxiety and stress. In fact, those who reported having conflicts with wives and children and answered "no" reported *twice* as much chest pain.[13]

Can Two Hearts Beat Better than One?

Two studies investigated the effect of marital status on survival after an initial heart attack. Both studies found that marriage, itself, serves as a protective factor for the heart.

Unmarried men had a significantly increased risk of death from heart disease and all other causes more than eight years after suffering a heart attack according to a study of 200 men in Sweden.[14] Similarly, another study investigated the short-term effect of living single after a heart attack. Six months after the initial event, those who were single or lived alone suffered almost twice as many heart attacks and deaths. The risk was independent of age, gender, severity of damage to the heart, drug treatment, or other confounding factors. One to four years after the fact, the risk did not change for these individuals.[15] However, yet to be identified is the specific aspect of being married (emotional, psychological, economical, social, or all of the above) that is affording the beneficial effect on heart health and survival.

Is Love in the Eye of the Beholder?

Apparently, it is the *perception* of support from others that is the key factor in soothing loneliness. Heart disease patients were asked to rate their perceived need for help with activities of daily living (for example, bathing and preparing foods). Perceptions of unmet needs were strongly associated with an increased risk of death and greater functional deterioration. Those individuals who reported needing "more help" had three times greater risk of dying; those reporting "much more help" had six times as much risk. As might be expected, individuals who were single or lived alone were less likely to perceive having adequate support.[16]

Emotional support, however, appears to be equally as important as instrumental support in predicting the survival of individuals with heart disease. A study looked at the impact of emotional support on the physical resilience of individuals hospitalized for an acute heart attack. The findings were as follows: (1) More than three times as many men and women who had no identifiable source of emotional support died in the hospital; (2) After six months, 53 percent of those with no source of support died. In comparison, death occurred in only 36 and 23 percent of those reporting one and two or more sources, respectively. Overall, after controlling for the influence of other factors such as severity of the heart attack, other illnesses, depression, or age, those men and women who reported having no emotional support has almost three times the mortality risk compared with those who had at least one source of support.[17]

Is Your Best Nonhuman Friend Saving Your Life?

There is a soft spot in our hearts for animal friends and their role in our lives. For some of us, it may be in this context that we experience true unconditional love. Animal friends create a safe emotional space for us to give and receive much needed physical affection. We perceive them as needing and appreciating us. They provide unlimited emotional support. Gaining the trust of an animal can be a very affirming experience. To use clinical jargon, animals provide "non-evaluative social support." All this, of course, is good for the heart. Perhaps the lesson we learn about loving and living from our nonhuman friends can carry over to our other relationships. A plaque which speaks to this issue reads: "God, help me to be the human being my dog thinks I am."

On a more scholarly note, there is a plethora of scientific research supporting the assertion that people who have animal friends are healthier than those who do not. For example, over six times as many individuals without the companionship of dogs died during a study of individuals who had sustained a heart attack and also had irregular heart-beats.[18] A year after being hospitalized with a heart attack or chest pain, only 6 percent of patients with pets died. In comparison, death occurred in 28 percent of patients who did not have pets.[19] Social interactions with animals can reduce your blood pressure.[20] Elderly people with pets required less physician services than their pet-less counterparts.[21]

In summary, we hope you take to heart that a positive perception of support (emotional, informational, and instrumental) during a period of high vulnerability (emotional or physical) is life preserving. In fact, the most effective intervention programs in reducing deaths after a heart attack make use of this therapeutic mechanism. The popularity of "support groups" is built on the notion that people need emotional intimacy to heal. However, in the same way that "social connectedness" can be sustaining, a heart's sense of loss may put your life at risk. This is not a surprise. Depression, with its ensuing feelings of psychological distress, emotional isolation and hopelessness, may be considered the ultimate form of disconnection.

> *The elderly with pets require less physician services than those without pets.*

Risk Factor #2: Depression and Hopelessness

On the issue of depression and heart disease, the research revealed that sub-clinical depression may pose an increased risk of heart disease. Ninety-three thousand women, ranging from 50 to 79 years of age, participated in this four-year study. At the onset of the study, 16 percent of the participants were assessed to be depressed; 12 percent reported a history of depression. Four years after the study began, depressed women (or those with a history of depression) had a *significantly increase risk of cardiovascular death and disease* than the control (0.79 versus 0.52 percent). But, the most dramatic finding was that *depression was an independent predictor* of cardiovascular death for women *without* a prior history of heart disease. The relative risk of cardiovascular death associated with depression was 1.5. This was the result after taking into account age, race, education, income, diabetes, hypertension, smoking, *high cholesterol requiring medication*, body mass index, and physical activity. Of note, the study found that taking antidepressant medication did not alter the associated risks.[22]

> *Depression creates a higher risk of heart problems regardless of cholesterol levels.*

Two other studies took the question a step further. They investigated the impact of the severity of depression on the risk heart disease. Unlike the first study, this one was composed entirely of elderly men.

In one study all 5,888 elderly participants were free of heart disease at the onset of the investigation. They were followed for six years during which time participants provided annual information on their depressive status. Results revealed that each 5-unit increase in depression score was associated with an odds ratio of 1.15 for the development of heart disease. This finding took into account age, race, sex, education, diabetes, hypertension, cigarette smoking, total cholesterol, triglycerides level, congestive heart failure, and physical activity. At the end of the six years, the cumulative depressive score was significantly associated with heart disease and total death. Participants with the *highest cumulative depressive scores had a 40 percent increased risk of heart disease and a 60 percent increased risk of death.*[23]

The second study asked the question: Can a major depressive episode increase the risk of a heart attack? This was a prospective study that lasted 13 years. Sixty-four heart attacks were reported among the 1,551 respondents who were free of heart disease at the onset of the study. The odds ratio for having a heart attack associated with a history of dysphoria (two weeks of sadness) was 2.07. *The odds ratio associated with a history of a major depressive episode was 4.54!* The relationship of depression and heart attacks was found to be independent of coronary risk factors.[24]

Additionally the following trends were revealed: (1) There was an increase in depression scores prior to a heart attack, stroke, or death;[25] and (2) In men, the recent onset of depression, but not chronic depression, was associated with an increase risk of cardiovascular mortality (relative risk 1.75).[26]

Lastly, according to a statistical study, losing someone dear to your heart may put *your* life at-risk. There was a 40 percent increase in the mortality rate of middle-aged widowers in the first six months following bereavement. More than half of all deaths were attributed to cardiovascular causes.[27] Another study showed that there was a relative risk of 14.3 that you would have a heart attack if you answered "yes" to the question: "During the past year, did you hear news of the death of a friend, relative or someone who was very significant in your life?"[28]

With the exception of the last two citations, it is not apparent from the data what factors triggered depression in the study participants. Moreover, all the studies involved middle-aged and elderly participants. Yet to be determined is whether results can be extrapolated to a younger population. These shortcomings do not diminish the powerful findings and poignant theme of the studies: Depression, short-lived or prolonged, quietly causing agony or overwhelming you with grief, can drive a stake through your heart.

Risk Factor #3: Anger and Anxiety

Stories abound of people who have "dropped dead" while clutching their hearts after receiving bad news. Similarly, there is the anecdote of the angry, red-faced, tense-body, screaming man who dies with clenched fists. Whether fiction or nonfiction, real life or on the movie screen, this scene has been ingrained in our minds so that we do not think to ask: "Can this be true?" Unfortunately, these anecdotes can, in fact, be substantiated by scientific research studies on the triggers of sudden heart attacks.

An analysis of possible triggers leading to a sudden heart attack revealed "emotional upset" as an identifiable cause in 18.4 percent of the cases.[29] Stressful life events occurred in 40 of 100 sudden death victims in the 24 hours preceding death. This study involved deaths that were so unexpected and sudden as to merit an autopsy by a coroner. Interestingly, factors such as very strenuous exercise, cigarette smoking, or the composition of the meal last ingested did not appear to affect the onset of the attack.[30]   These studies, unfortunately, do not define clearly the nature of the "emotional upset."

In order to put in context the effect of negative emotions on the heart, consider this: Violent verbal quarrels and unusual mental stress were two of the three most frequently reported triggers preceding chest pain. The other trigger was exceptional heavy physical work.[31]

What Does Anger Have To Do With It?

Hostility, cynicism, and anger are behaviors that are associated with a greater risk of cardiovascular disease.[32] This has been well documented in long-term studies with individuals who exhibit these behaviors as part of their personality (often referred to "Type A" individuals). Also, a review of more than 45 studies concluded that hostility was a key factor in disease. Hostility was equal to or greater in magnitude to the traditional risk factors for heart disease (i.e., high blood pressure and cholesterol levels).[33] However, even a single episode of anger has also been demonstrated to trigger a heart attack.

In a study of 1,623 patients (520 women) who survived a heart attack, episodes of anger immediately preceded and appeared to trigger the onset of a heart attack. Thirty-nine patients clearly identified an episode of anger in the two hours before the onset of the attack. Arguments with family members accounted as the most frequent cause of anger in 25 percent of those interviewed. Overall, data revealed a relative risk of 2.3 that an attack can occur after an episode of anger.[34]

Can You be Literally 'Scared to Death'?

A prospective study was done on the effect of anxiety (phobic anxiety) on the risk of heart disease. The study included 33,999 men, ranging in age from 42 to 77, who were free of diagnosed heart disease at the onset of the study. Data revealed a 3.01 age-adjusted relative risk of death due to anxiety. Highest phobic anxiety related to sudden deaths more than non-sudden death. There was a dose-response gradient of the association between fear and death. This means that the risk was greatest among those who reported the highest levels of phobic anxiety, lowest among those with the least.[35]

Summary

It is the hope in sharing these studies to alert the reader regarding the hazards of living a life of emotional isolation, grief, and strife. But, it is not until the "heart," your seat of emotion, embraces this message that wisdom comes. Perhaps this reading has offered you an opportunity to resolve to make changes at the most basic level of your health — the level that governs your emotions — your psyche.

Whether your interest is preventing heart disease or you are undergoing rehabilitation, with every choice you make, ask yourself: Is this in the best interest of my heart? Let your broken heart lead you to a path of wisdom; thus, may you live a joyous and fulfilling life.

Healing a Broken Heart

General suggestions for creating heart health.

The antidote for loneliness:
- Consider cognitive or behavioral counseling to address issues of emotional intimacy that may be keeping you from engaging with others.

- Make friends with another species: Adopt an animal – any kind, but preferably one that needs you and you can pet.

- Join an organization or group with emotional warmth.

- Join a cultural or ethnic society.

- Join a spiritual community such as a church or meditation group with whom you can congregate with regularly.

- Build a community of kindred spirit by creating or joining an interest group.

- Volunteer to do community service that involves helping people in need.

- Get yourself a good listening friend and confidant and cherish the relationship.

- Find a spiritual-director or counselor with whom you can engage in discussion about spiritual and emotions issues.

- Consider joining a "support group." As discussed, support comes in different forms, for example, emotional, instrumental, or informational. Identify the kind of support you are lacking and find a group that fills this need.

- Cultivate a loving relationship with your significant other. Learn to understand what makes *them* feel loved. Speak their emotional language.

- Make it a point to be open about your emotional and physical needs. Learn to understand what makes *you* feel loved. Teach others your emotional language.

The antidote for depression:
- Find yourself a teacher and begin the practice of meditation (do this now!).

- Cultivate the practice of meditation as if your life depended on it.

- Read inspirational books, watch uplifting movies, surround yourself with positive people.

- Breathe in nature.

- Join a prayer group for emotional healing.

The antidote for anger:
- Find yourself a teacher and begin the practice of meditation (do this now!)

- Cultivate the practice of meditation as if your life depended on it.

- Consider cognitive or behavior therapy.

- Consider learning biofeedback.

- Find laughter in every day. Laughter is good medicine.

* 10 *
PUTTING IT ALL TOGETHER

A man has a heart attack. Which of the following factors will most accurately predict a second heart attack in the next six months?
   A. Whether he continues to smoke
   B. Whether he is depressed
   C. Whether his cholesterol remains elevated
   D. Whether he follows up with a cardiologist
   E. Whether he can tango with a mango

The factor that most accurately predicts a second heart-attack is depression. Emotional factors play a huge role in heart disease. Unfortunately, these factors have been ignored until recently. Depression is such a strong risk factor that some cardiologists started to routinely prescribe antidepressants after an initial heart attack in the late 1990s. However, studies later showed that antidepressants did not help. Even though the association between the recurrence of a heart-attack and depression was still there, treating a depressive emotional state with drugs did not prevent a second heart-attack.

Emotional wellness, stress, diet, and exercise play a larger role in preventing heart disease than monitoring your cholesterol. Let us tabulate some of these factors and rank them in relation to the amount of risk reduction cited in clinical studies.

Percent Reduction in Cardiovascular Risk

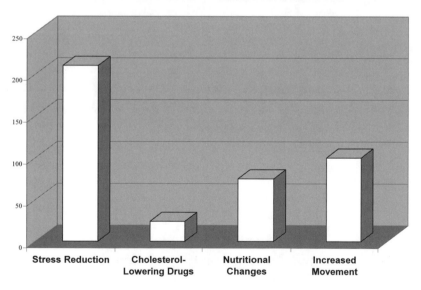

As you can see from the graph, the impact of cholesterol-lowering drugs pales in comparison to what can be attained through lifestyle changes. In fact, as we have already pointed out, the cholesterol-lowering drugs probably prevent heart disease by mechanisms other than reducing cholesterol.

The new generation of statin drugs poses problems yet to be determined. Their effect after decades of continuous use is yet unknown. Initially, laboratory testing showed that these drugs induced cancer in rats.[1] Clinicians reserved their use only for patients who were not likely to live long enough to develop cancer. Their current use, however, has become more liberal. In the wake of one blockbuster drug after another producing harmful effects with long-term use, it seems hard to justify experimenting with the statin drugs on otherwise healthy people. Here is the main point: You can benefit much more by changing factors under your control than from taking drugs. These changes will not cost you money. Their side effects are only positive and life-enriching.

> *By changing factors under your control, you can benefit much more than from taking drugs.*

Needless to say, if you have an existing heart condition, drug use may be necessary. If that is the case, it would be best to avoid those drugs that easily cross the blood-brain barrier: atorvastatin (Lipitor), lovastatin (Mevacor), and simvastatin

(Zocor). *Let us underscore that incorporating the recommended life-style changes can only enhance the effects of any drug you may take.*

If we assume that lifestyle changes are cumulative in their effect, let us graphically look at what happens if you make more than one change:

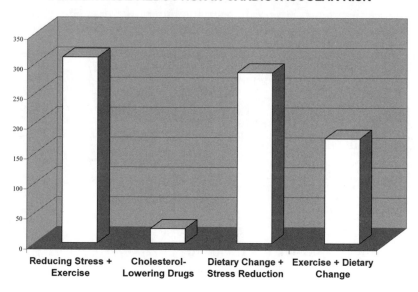

PERCENTAGE REDUCTION IN CARDIOVASCULAR RISK

Finally, what happens if we put it all together? That is, what if you start meditating, make appropriate dietary changes, improve your relationships, exercise, and decrease stress and hostility. Then the comparison looks like this:

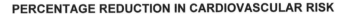

PERCENTAGE REDUCTION IN CARDIOVASCULAR RISK

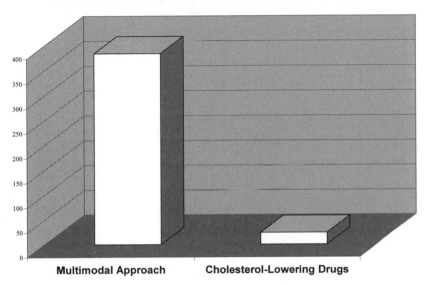

Multimodal Approach   **Cholesterol-Lowering Drugs**

Putting it all together translates into a huge potential reduction in your risk of heart and artery disease. Unfortunately, there is yet to be a study where all these protective lifestyle changes were incorporated into a single program for a large number of men and women. Thus, medical science has yet to fully appreciate the potential benefits derived from these lifestyle changes. It may be that these changes work in a synergistic manner, so their effect may be multiplicative rather than simply additive.

One Bold Individual

One bold individual, however, aggressively undertook the implementation of lifestyle changes in treating severely ill individuals. While the studies involved small numbers of people, the outcomes were revolutionary. Until Dr. Dean Ornish undertook his studies of individuals with known heart disease, few in the medical community thought that lifestyle changes alone could considerably affect coronary artery disease.

Ornish studied individuals with known coronary artery disease. These individuals had come to the attention of the medical community because their heart disease was sufficiently advanced to produce symptoms — usually angina or the squeezing sensation of chest pain. This group was offered the option of participating in a study that tried to prevent heart problems without drugs or surgery. They were randomized to either an intensive lifestyle change program or to a control group that received usual medical care. Those who were in the lifestyle change program participated in a program that included meditation, counseling, low-fat vegetarian diet, exercise, and smoking cessation.

Ornish thought that his program would help prevent further clogging of the arteries. He planned to monitor the subjective symptomatic improvement of his patients. Additionally, patients underwent heart studies where the amount of clogging of the arteries can be visualized with a special dye (catheterization of the heart). This would provide objective information about their level of heart disease.

The results of his study were impressive. For the first time in the history of medical science, Ornish demonstrated conclusively that the progression of atherosclerosis could be stopped without drugs. However, the more astounding revelation was that drugfree interventions could actually *reverse* heart disease.

After five years, the control group showed an absolute increase in narrowing of the arteries of 11.8 percent. On the other hand, the lifestyle change group showed a *reduction* in arterial narrowing of 3.1 percent. More importantly, the risk of a cardiac event, such as heart attack or the onset of angina, was 147 percent less in the experimental group than in the control group (relative risk of 2.47).[2]

The results of his program were so impressive that after reproducing the results from the initial "experiment," insurance companies began to pay for the intensive lifestyle education and counseling. After all, this program was only one-fourth the cost of bypass surgery. The number of individuals who suffered recurring heart attacks was no greater than with surgery.

Pritikin

Lifestyle interventions that combine multiple modalities were also studied in the 1980s by Nathan Pritikin. Participants in the Pritikin program underwent 26 days of physical activity and dietary intervention at a residential facility. Vegetarian, buffet-style meals allowed unrestricted eating. The only dietary limitation was a 3-ounce portion of animal protein (fish or fowl) when it was served. Meals were low-fat (10-15 percent of calories) and low-protein (15-20 percent of calories). Unrefined carbohydrates composed the major source of calories.

All participants completed a medical history, physical examination, and a graded treadmill stress test prior to starting the program. Based on these factors, subjects were given an individualized aerobic exercise program and "heart-rate limit." This program consisted, for example, of daily treadmill walking at their training heart rate for 45-60 minutes. As a result of the Pritikin program, the majority of participants were able to eliminate their cardiac and blood pressure medications. Additionally, the program dramatically reduced the need for cardiac bypass surgery.[3]

Ornish popularized the field of lifestyle medicine. Few know, however, that the essence of his program was motivated by his contact with the East. His book *Love and Intimacy* (1995) reveals his journey.

As a student of yoga and meditation, Ornish experienced firsthand the potential benefits that Oriental wisdom could offer. In the United States, the wisdom of the East is gradually becoming more appreciated. Most people do not know, however, that yoga and meditation are two prongs of a comprehensive medical system called Ayurveda.

Ayurveda is the primary care for approximately 800 million people in India and southeast Asia. The cornerstone of this system is the interaction of mind and body, as well as the importance of diet. In addition, it has a robust herbal *materia medica* with more than 5,000 plants. It offers techniques for lifestyle change and for altering the inner awareness of the individual, making heart-healthy behaviors easy.

Ayurveda understands that a rich diet, high in sugar, oils, and/or meats, can create the buildup of undigested and unutilized materials. This concept is very similar to the Western medical concept of advanced glycosylation end-products. This toxic buildup can create inflammation and affect the function of the immune system. Ayurveda understands that food can be inflammatory, and it provides knowledge of how to counteract an inflammatory state with the use of certain foods and spices.

Dr. Robert Schneider has incorporated Ayurveda into the treatment of heart disease. The small population of African-Americans in his study were offered Ayurvedic knowledge about nutrition, along with herbal prescriptions, such as antioxidants like Amrit Kalash. They were also taught Transcendental Meditation. However, no large-scale study has been undertaken to utilize the full knowledge and wisdom of the ancient medical systems in preventing heart disease. The future of medicine may very well see Ayurvedic and Chinese medicine as the mainstay of outpatient medicine and prevention. The potential for research and for cure is there to be explored and may far exceed all expectations.

Keeping a Healthy Heart

It will take time for the American public to make the shift away from laboratory medicine toward natural medical systems like Ayurveda or Chinese medicine. In the meantime, if you would like to check external measures of heart health, we recommendation you present these to your doctor. All of these laboratory tests are commonly available at most labs:

- Homocysteine — A measure of the toxic metabolite of amino acids

- C-reactive protein (CRP) — A measure of general inflammation in the body

- Fasting Insulin — A measure of whether the body is overloaded and resisting the normal effects of insulin when elevated

- Vitamin B12, Folate — Important vitamins in converting homocysteine to nontoxic amino acids

- Vitamin C — Low levels may cause a decrease in elasticity of arteries and an indirect increase in homocysteine levels

- Triglycerides — A measure of excess intake of fats and sugars

It may be valuable to find out your blood levels of these substances before starting your lifestyle changes. Levels can be rechecked three months later. However, these laboratory values are not necessary for you to have in order to benefit from the changes recommended in this book. These values will all improve if you take the suggestions we have given in the second half of the book. But, more importantly, the benefits of engaging in the recommended lifestyle changes will be experienced as a sense of overall wellness.

Finally, we are often asked whether anyone should bother to measure cholesterol, if it is of minimal importance in heart health. Lipid profiles can be useful as a screening test to find those individuals with a genetic defect in cholesterol metabolism. Beyond this, an annual check is not needed for most people. Some experts recommend testing cholesterol once every five years. We would agree with that more conservative approach, unless you have one of the genetic problems in your family.

Avert Magic Bullets

If you select the laboratory medicine route to gauge your health status, do not be fooled by the magic bullet theory. Many people ignore those low-tech things they can do to promote heart health in favor of taking a pill (natural or synthetic). Unfortunately, sometimes those who are wary of the drugs fall into the same mistaken line of thinking by taking "natural" pills.

Nutritional supplements are peddled with equal fervor as magic bullets. Currently available are such supplements as red rice yeast (a natural form of the cholesterol-lowering drug lovastatin) and policolsanol, another statin-like supplement that is derived from sugarcane wax. Policolsanol is used in Cuba by allopathic physicians as an inexpensive statin drug. It works to lower cholesterol and is available as a nutritional supplement in this country. These supplements have their place, particularly in individuals with heart disease who cannot afford expensive statin drugs. But as with other magic bullets, these "natural" supplements detract from the real benefits of focusing on a heart-healthy lifestyle.

Keeping a healthy heart involves more than looking at a number on a lab report. By focusing so exclusively on cholesterol, the prevention efforts of the medical community have created a myth that is hard to eradicate — the myth that if you watch your cholesterol your heart will be healthy. Like so much in life, heart health is more complicated than that. Unfortunately at this point, you cannot rely only on the medical profession to offer you knowledge on how to cultivate heart health. While many doctors know the profound results that lifestyle modification offers, they are not very effective at helping patients with this most important aspect of health promotion. In fact, one study notes that 51 percent of primary care physicians do not even suggest dietary modification before starting drug therapy for elevated cholesterol. Twenty-nine percent do not counsel patients on diet after starting drugs.[4] This over-reliance on the power of the magic bullet has been responsible for the lack of progress in cardiovascular health in the United States.

The good news, though, is that the most important interventions and the most important means to a healthy heart are in your control. You do not have to go to a doctor, a pharmacist, or a hospital in order to make dramatic reductions in your risk of heart disease.

The Need of the Time

The belief that cholesterol alone causes heart disease must be laid to rest. We do not need another scapegoat or another laboratory value by which to measure our health. What is the need of the time? Our society needs to respect the inner wisdom of the human mind and body. In understanding the depths of consciousness and the profound interactions between mind and body, the key to profound change can be found. This knowledge will affect the health of individuals, as well as society as a whole.

The myth of cholesterol has distracted us from making real advances in heart health and preventive medicine. The consequences of this misconception are being reaped each year in terms of more and more heart disease and suffering. By dispelling this myth, we aim to challenge those who want true heart health to reclaim their power to create their own health. No pill can substitute for a healthy lifestyle. And that lifestyle must include a healthy diet, healthy movement, and mental and emotional well-being. Without myths, we can live healthy, happy lives, experiencing each day fully, with vigor and whole-heartedness. After all, it is what we deserve.

RESOURCES

Important Books

Erasmus, Udo. *Fats that Heal, Fats that Kill.* (Burnaby, BC, Canada: Alive Books, 1993).

Graveline D. *Lipitor: Thief of Memory.* (Haverford, PA: Infinity Publishing Co., 2004).

McCully KS, McCully M. *The Heart Revolution.* (New York: HarperCollins, 1999).

Pert C. *Molecules of Emotion.* (New York: Scribner, 1997).

Ravnskov U, *The Cholesterol Myths.* (Washington, DC: New Trends Publishing, 2000).

Roth R. *Transcendental Meditation.* (New York: Donald I. Fine, Inc., 1994).

Sanson G. *The Myth of Osteoporosis.* (Ann Arbor, Michigan: MCD Century Publications, 2003).

Nutrition Books

Hospadar M. *Heaven's Banquet.* (New York: Penquin Putnam, 1999).

Kesten D. *The Healing Secrets of Food.* (Novato, California: New World Library, 2001).

Morningstar A. *Ayurvedic Cooking for Westerners.* (Twin Lakes, Wisconsin: Lotus Press, 1995).

Important Web Sites

- Transcendental Meditation: http://www. tm.org
- Scientific research (Public Medline):   http://www.ncbi.nlm.nih.gov/entrez/
- Clinically-oriented medical research: http://www.uptodate.com

REFERENCES

Chapter 2

[1]Murray RK, Branner DK, Mayes PA, Rodwell VW. *Harper's Biochemistry, 21 Ed.* (East Norwalk, Connecticut: Appleton & Lange, 1988), 241.

[2]*Ibid*, 241.

[3]*Ibid.*

[4]Graveline, D. *Lipitor: Thief of Memory.* (Haverford, PA: Infinity Publishing Co., 2004).

[5]Pfrieger B. Brain research discovers bright side of ill-famed molecule. *Science*, 9 November 2001.

[6]Wagstaff LR, et al. Statin-associated memory loss: Analysis of 60 case reports and review of literature. *Pharmacotherapy.* 2003; 23(7):871-880.

[7]Lazarou J, Pomeranz BH, Corey PN. Incidence of adverse drug reactions in hospitalized patients: A meta-analysis of prospective studies. *Journal of the American Medical Association.* 1998 Apr 15; 279(15):1200-5.

[8]Wallach J. *Interpretation of Diagnostic Tests.* (Little, Brown and Company, Inc., 1996), 478-51.

[9]Gotto AM, Paolett R, Eds. *The Atherosclerosis Reviews*, Vol. 11. (New York, NY: Raven Press, 1983), 157-246.

Chapter 3

[1]Kannel WB. High-density lipoproteins: Epidemiologic profile and risks of coronary artery disease. *American Journal of Cardiology.* 1983; 52:9B.

[2]Ravskov U. *The Cholesterol Myths.* (Washington, DC: New Trends Publishing, 2000).

[3]Medalie JH, et al. Five-year myocardial infarction incidence – II. Association of single variables to age and birthplace. *Journal of Chronic Diseases.* 1973; 26:329-349.

[4]Ravskov U. *The Cholesterol Myths.* (Washington, DC: New Trends Publishing, 2000), 123.

[5]Lande KE, Sperry WM. Human atherosclerosis in relation to the cholesterol content of the blood serum. *Archives of Pathology.* 1936; 22:301-12.

[6]Mathur KS, et al. Serum cholesterol and atherosclerosis in man. *Circulation.* 1961; 23:847-52.

[7]Paterson JC, Armstrong R, Armstrong EC. Serum lipid levels and the severity of coronary and cerebral atherosclerosis in adequately nourished men, 60 to 69 years of age. *Circulation.* 1963; 27:229-36.

[8]Feinleib M, et al. The relation of antemortem characteristics to cardiovascular findings at necropsy. The Framingham Study. *Atherosclerosis.* 1979; 34:145-57.

[9]Kita T, et al. Probucol prevents the progression of atherosclerosis in Watanabbe heritable hyperlipidemic rabbits: An animal model for familial hypercholesterolemia. *Proceedings of the National Academy of Science.* 1987; 84:5928.

[10]Phillips RL, Kuzman JW, Beeson WL, Lots T. Influence of selection versus lifestyle on risk of fatal cancer and cardiovascular disease among Seventh-Day Adventists. *American Journal of Epidemiology.* 1980; 112:296-314.

[11]Stephens NG, Parsons A, Schofield PM, Kelly F, Cheeseman K, Mitchinson MJ. Randomised controlled trial of vitamin E in patients with coronary disease: Cambridge Heart Antioxidant Study (CHAOS). *Lancet.* 1996 Mar 23; 347(9004):781-6.

[12]Sharma HM, Hanna AN, Kaufman EM, Newman HAI. Inhibition of human low-density lipoprotein oxidation in-vitro by Maharishi Ayurveda herbal mix. *Pharmacology, Biochemistry and Behavior.* 1992; 43:1175-82.

[13]Dogra J, Grover N, Kumar P, Aneja N. Indigenous free-radical scavenger MAK-4 and MAK-5 in angina pectoris. Is it placebo. *Journal of the Association of Physicians in India.* 1994; 42(6):466-7.

[14]Kip KE, Marroquin OC, Kelly DE, Johnson BD, Kelsey SF, Shaw LF, Rogers WJ, Reiss SE. Clinical importance of obesity versus the metabolic syndrome in cardiovascular risk in women: A report from the Women's Ischemic Syndrome Evaluation (WISE) Study. *Circulation*. 2004 Feb 17; 109(6):706-13.

Chapter 4

[1]Anderson KM, Castelli WP, Levy D. Cholesterol and mortality. 30 years of follow-up from the Framingham Study. *Journal of the American Medical Association*. 1987; 257:2176-2180.

[2]Bartlett DL, Steele JB. *Critical Condition*, (New York: Doubleday, 2004), 252.

[3]Greenland P, Knoll MD, Stamler J, et al. Major risk factors as antecedents of fatal and nonfatal coronary heart disease events. *Journal of the American Medical Association*. 2003 Aug 20; 290(7): 891-897.

[4]*Ibid.*

[5]Ford ES, Mokdad AH, Giles WH, Mensah GA. Serum total choelsterol concentrations and awareness, treatment and control of hypercholesterolemia among US adults: findings from the National Health and Nutrition Examination Survey, 1999 to 2000. *Circulation*. 2003 May 6; 107(17): 2185-2189.

[6]*Op. cit.*

[7]See Wallach J. *Interpretation of Diagnostic Tests*. (Little, Brown and Company, Inc., 1996).

Chapter 5

[1]Report from the Committee of Principal Investigators. A co-operative trial in the primary prevention of ischaemic heart disease using clofibrate. *British Heart Journal*. 1978; 40:1069.

[2]Report of the Committee of Principal Investigators. W.H.O. cooperative trial on primary prevention of ischaemic heart disease using clofibrate to lower serum cholesterol: mortality follow-up. *Lancet*. 1980; 2:379.

[3]The Lipid Research Clinics Coronary Primary Prevention Trial results. I. Reduction in incidence of coronary heart disease. *Journal of the American Medical Association*. 1984; 251:351.

[4]The Lipid Research Clinics Coronary Primary Prevention Trial results. II. The relationship of reduction in incidence of coronary heart disease to cholesterol lowering. *Journal of the American Medical Association*. 1984; 251:365.

[5]Frick MH, Elo O, Haapa K, et al. Helsinki Heart Study: Primary prevention trial with gemfibrozil in middle-aged men with dyslipidemia. Safety of treatment, changes in risk factors, and incidence of coronary heart disease. *New England Journal of Medicine.* 1987; 317:1237.

[6]Shepherd J, Cobbe SM, Ford I, et al. Prevention of coronary heart disease with pravastatin in men with hypercholesterolemia. *New England Journal of Medicine.* 1995; 333:1301.

[7]Downs JR, Clearfield M, Weis S, et al for the AFCAPS/TexCAPS Research Group. Primary prevention of acute coronary events with lovastatin in men and women with average cholesterol levels: Results of AFCAPS/TexCAPS. *Journal of the American Medical Association.* 1998; 279:1615.

[8]Sever PS, Dahlof B, Poulter NR, et al. Prevention of coronary and stroke events with atorvastatin in hypertensive patients who have average or lower-than-average cholesterol concentrations, in the Anglo-Scandinavian Cardiac Outcomes Trial-Lipid Lowering Arm (ASCOT-LLA): a multicentre randomised controlled trial. *Lancet.* 2003; 361:1149.

[9]Ravnskov U. *The Cholesterol Myths.* (Washington, DC: NewTrends Publishing, 2000), 205.

[10]Watts GF, Lewis B, Brunt JN, et al. Effects on coronary artery disease of lipid-lowering diet or diet plus cholestyramine in the St. Thomas' Atherosclerosis Regression Study (STARS). *Lancet.* 1992; 339:563.

[11]de Lorgeril M, et al. Mediterranean alpha-linolenic acid-rich diet in secondary prevention of coronary heart disease. *Lancet.* 1994; 343:1454.

[12]Randomised trial of cholesterol lowering in 4,444 patients with coronary heart disease: the Scandinavian Simvastatin Survival Study (4S). *Lancet.* 1994; 334:1383.

[13]Pedersen TR, Wihelmsen L, Faergeman O, et al. Follow-up study of patients randomized in the Scandinavian Simvastatin Survival Study (4S). *American Journal of Cardiology.* 2000; 86:257.

[14]Pedersen TR, Olsson AG, Faergeman O, et al. for the Scandinavian Simvastatin Survival Study Group. Lipoprotein changes and reduction in the incidence of major coronary heart disease events in the Scandinavian Simvastatin Survival Study (4S). *Circulation.* 1998; 97:1453.

[15]Prevention of cardiovascular events and death with pravastatin in patients with coronary heart disease and a broad range of initial cholesterol levels. The Long-Term Intervention with Pravastatin in Ischaemic Disease (LIPID) Study Group. *New England Journal of Medicine.* 1998; 339:1349.

[16]MRC/BHF Heart Protection Study of cholesterol lowering with simvastatin in 20,536 high-risk individuals: a randomised placebo-controlled trial. *Lancet.* 2002; 360:7.

[17]Schwartz GG, Olsson AG, Ezekowitz MD, et al. Effects of atorvastatin on early recurrent ischemic events in acute coronary syndromes. The MIRACL Study: A randomized controlled trial. *Journal of the American Medical Association.* 2001; 285:1711.

Chapter 6

Lindethal J, Myers J, Pepper M. Smoking, psychological status, and stress. *Social Science Medicine.* 1972; 6:583.

[2]Dimsdale JE, Herd JA. Variability of plasma lipids in response to emotional arousal. *Psychosomatic Medicine.* 1982; 44:413.

[3]Rahe R, Rubin R, Arthur R. The three investigators study: Serum uric acid, cholesterol and cortisol variability during stresses of everyday life. *Psychosomatic Medicine.* 1974; 36:258.

[4]*Ibid.*

[5]Dimsdale JE, Herd JA, Hartley LH. Epinephrine mediated increases in plasma cholesterol. *Psychosomatic Medicine.* 1983; 45:227.

[6]Henry JP, Ely DL, Stephens PM, et al. The role of psychosocial factors in the development of arteriosclerosis in CBA mice: Observations on the heart, kidney, and aorta. *Arteriosclerosis.* 1971; 14:203.

[7]Strawn WB, Bondjers G, Kaplan JR, et al. Endothelial dysfunction in response to psychosocial stress in monkeys. *Circulation Research.* 1991; 68:1270.

[8]Ross R. The pathogenesis of atherosclerosis: A perspective for the 1990s. *Nature.* 1993; 362:801.

[9]Ghiadoni L, Donald AE, Cropley M, et al. Mental stress induces transient endothelial dysfunction in humans. *Circulation.* 2000; 102:2473.

[10]Spieker LE, Hurlimann D, Ruschitzka F, et al. Mental stress induces prolonged endothelial dysfunction via endothelin-A receptors. *Circulation.* 2002; 105:2817.

[11]*Ibid.*

[12]*Ibid.*

[13]Cardillo C, Kilcoyne CM, Cannon RO, et al. Impairment of the nitric oxide-mediated vasodilator response to mental stress in hypertensive, but not in hypercholesterolemic patients. *Journal of the American College of Cardiology.* 1998; 32:1207.

[14]Haft JI, Arkel YS. Effect of emotional stress on platelet aggregation in humans. *Chest.* 1976; 70:501.

[15]Wagner CT, Kroll MH, Chow TW, et al. Epinephrine and shear stress synergistically induce platelet aggregation via a mechanism that partially bypasses vWF-GPIB interactions. *Biorheology.* 1996; 33:209.

[16]Roux SP, Sakariassen KS, Turitto VT, et al. Effect of aspirin and epinephrine on experimentally induced thrombogenesis in dogs. *Arteriosclerosis Thrombogenesis.* 1991; 11:1182.

[17]Henry JP, Meehan JP, Stephens PM. The use of psychosocial stimuli to induce prolonged systolic hypertension in mice. *Psychosomatic Medicine.* 1967; 29:408.

[18]Krantz DS, Manuck SB. Acute psychophysiologic reactivity and risk of cardiovascular disease: A review and methodologic critique. *Psychology Bulletins.* 1984; 96:435.

[19]Chang PP, Ford DE, Meoni LA, et al. Anger in young men and subsequent premature cardiovascular disease. The Precursors study. *Archives of Internal Medicine.* 2002; 162:901.

[20]Kivimaki M, Leino-Arjas P, Luukkonen R, et al. Work stress and risk of cardiovascular mortality: prospective cohort study of industrial employees. *British Medical Journal.* 2002; 325:857.

[21]Sesso HD, Kawachi I, Vokonas PS, et al. Depression and the risk of coronary heart disease in the Normative Aging study. *American Journal Cardiology.* 1998; 82:851.

[22]*Ibid.*

[23]Kawachi I, Sparrow D, Spiro A 3rd, et al. A prospective study of anger and coronary heart disease. The Normative Aging Study. *Circulation.* 1996; 94:2090.

[24]Siegman AW, Kubzansky LD, Kawachi I, et al. A prospective study of dominance and coronary heart disease in the Normative Aging Study. *American Journal Cardiology.* 2000; 86:145.

[25]Orme-Johnson DM, Medical Care Utilization and the Transcendental Meditation Program. *Psychosomatic Medicine.* 1987; 49:493-507.

[26]Herron RE, Hillis SL, Mandarino JV, Orme-Johnson DW, Walton KG. The impact of the Transcendental Meditation Program on government payments to physicians in Quebec. *American Journal of Health Promotion.* 1996 Jan-Feb; 10(3):208-216.

[27]Herron RE, Hillis SL. The impact of the Transcendental Meditation Program on government payments to physicians in Quebec: an update. *American Journal of Health Promotion.* 2000 May-Jun; 14(5):284-291.

[28]Schneider TH, Staggers F, Alexander CN, et al. A randomised controlled trial of stress reduction for hypertension in older African Americans. *Hypertension.* 1995 Nov; 26(5):820-827.

[29]Alexander CN, Schneider RH, Staggers F, et al. Trial of stress reduction for hypertension in older African Americans. II. Sex and risk subgroup analysis. *Hypertension.* 1996 Aug; 28(2):228-237.

[30]Schneider RH, Nidich SI, Salerno JW, Sharma HM, et al. Lower lipid peroxide levels in practitioners of the Transcendental Meditation Program. *Psychosomatic Medicine.* 1998 Jan-Feb; 60(1):38-41.

[31]Orme-Johnson DW, Walton KG. All approaches to preventing and reversing the effects of stress are not the same. *American Journal of Health Promotion.* 1998; 12(5):297-299.

Chapter 7

Fleming RM, The effect of high-protein diets on coronary blood flow. *Angiology.* 2000 Oct; 51(1):817-826.

[2]McCully KS, McCully M. *The Heart Revolution* (New York: HarperCollins, 1999), 12.

[3]*Ibid.*, 81.

[4]*Ibid.* 58-68.

[5]Roberts CK, Barnard RJ. Effects of exercise and diet on chronic disease. *Journal of Applied Physiology* 2005; 98: 3-30. citing the work by Campbell, Parpia and Chen:

Campbell TC, Parpia B, Chen J. Diet, lifestyle, and the etiology of coronary artery disease: the Cornell China study. *American Journal of Cardiology* 1998; 82:18T-21T.

[6]Gotto AM, Paolett R, Eds. *The Atherosclerosis Reviews.* Vol. 11 (New York: Raven Press, 1983), 157-246.

[7]de Lorgeril M, et al. Mediterranean alpha-linolenic acid-rich diet in secondary prevention of coronary heart disease. *The Lancet.* 1994; 343:1454-1459m.

[8]Hu FB, Stampfer MJ, Manson JE, et al. Dietary fat intake and the risk of coronary heart disease in women. *New England Journal of Medicine.* 1997; 337:1491.

[9]Din JN, Newby DE, Flapna AD. Omega-3 fatty acids and cardiovascular disease — fishing for a natural treatment. *British Medical Journal.* 2004; 328:30.

[10]Alexander JC, Valli VE, Chanin BE. Biological observations from feeding heated corn oil and heated peanut oil to rats. *Journal of Toxicology and Environmental Health.* 1987; 21:295-309.

[11]Gillman MW, Cupples LA, Millen BE, et al. Inverse associations of dietary fat with development of ischemic stroke in men. *Journal of the American Medical Association.* 1997; 278:2145.

[12]Mozaffarian D, Rimm EB, Herington DM. Dietary fats, carbohydrate, and progression of coronary atherosclerosis in postmenopausal women. *American Journal of Clinical Nutrition.* 2004 Nov; 80(5):1175-84.

[13]Gupta R, Prakash H. Association of dietary ghee intake with coronary heart disease and risk factor prevalence in rural males. *Journal of the Indian Medical Association.* 1997 Mar; 95(3):67-9, 83.

[14]Willet WC. Diet and health: What should we eat? *Science.* 1994; 264:532.

[15]Ravnskov U. *Cholesterol Myths.* (Washington, DC: New Trends Publishing, 2003), 230.

[16]Reaven GM. Banting lecture 1988. Role of insulin resistance in human disease. *Diabetes.* 1988 Dec; 37(12):1595-607.

[17]DeFronzo RA, Ferrannini E. Insulin resistance. A multifaceted syndrome responsible for NIDDM, obesity, hypertension, dyslipidemia, and atherosclerotic cardiovascular disease. *Diabetes Care.* 1991 Mar; 14(3):173-94.

[18]Lindsay RS, Howard BV. Cardiovascular risk associated with the metabolic syndrome. *Current Diabetes Reports.* 2004 Feb; 4(1):63-8.

[19]Festa A, D'Agostino R Jr, Tracy RP, Haffner SM. Elevated levels of acute-phase proteins and plasminogen activator inhibitor-1 predict the development of type 2 diabetes: the insulin resistance atherosclerosis study. *Diabetes.* 2002 Apr; 51(4):1131-7.

[20]Pradhan AD, Manson JE, Rifai N, Buring JE, Ridker PM. C-reactive protein, interleukin 6, and risk of developing type 2 diabetes mellitus. *Journal of the American Medical Association.* 2001 Jul 18; 286(3):327-34.

[21]Ridker PM, Buring JE, Cook NR, Rifai N. C-reactive protein, the metabolic syndrome, and risk of incident cardiovascular events: an 8-year follow-up of 14,719 initially healthy American women. *Circulation.* 2003 Jan 28; 107(3):391-7.

[22]Festa A, D'Agostino R Jr, Howard G, Mykkanen L, Tracy RP, Haffner SM. Chronic subclinical inflammation as part of the insulin resistance syndrome: the Insulin Resistance Atherosclerosis Study (IRAS). *Circulation.* 2000 Jul 4; 102(1):42-7.

[23]Sattar N, Gaw A, Scherbakova O, et al. Metabolic syndrome with and without C-reactive protein as a predictor of coronary heart disease and diabetes in the West of Scotland Coronary Prevention Study. *Circulation.* 2003 Jul 29; 108(4):414-9. Epub 2003 Jul 14.

[24]Lakka HM, Laaksonen DE, Lakka TA, et al. The metabolic syndrome and total and cardiovascular disease mortality in middle-aged men. *Journal of the American Medical Association.* 2002 Dec 4; 288(21):2709-16.

[25]Girman CJ, Rhodes T, Mercuri M, et al. The metabolic syndrome and risk of major coronary events in the Scandinavian Simvastatin Survival Study (4S)

and the Air Force/Texas Coronary Atherosclerosis Prevention Study (AFCAPS/TexCAPS). *American Journal of Cardiology.* 2004 Jan 15; 93(2):136-41.

[26]Kip KE, Marroquin OC, Kelley DE, Johnson BD, et al. Clinical importance of obesity versus the metabolic syndrome in cardiovascular risk in women: a report from the Women's Ischemia Syndrome Evaluation (WISE) study. *Circulation.* 2004 Feb 17; 109(6):706-13.

[27]Yudkin J, Eias O. Dietary Sucrose and Oestradiol Concentration in Young Men. *Annuals of Nutrition and Metabolism.* 1988; 32(2):53-55.

[28]Liu S, Manson, JE, Buring JE, et al. Relation between a diet with a high glycemic load and plasma concentrations of high-sensitivity C-reactive protein in middle-aged women. *American Journal of Clinical Nutrition.* 2002 Mar; 75(3):492-498.

[29]Erasmus, Udo. *Fats that Heal, Fats that Kill.* (Burnaby, BC, Canada: Alive Books, 1993), 69.

Chapter 8

Roberts CK, Barnard RJ. Effects of exercise and diet on chronic disease. *Journal of Applied Physiology.* 2005; 98: 3-30.

[2]*Ibid.*

[3]Wegge JK, Roberts CK, Ngo TH, Barnard RJ. Effect of diet and exercise intervention on inflammatory and adhesion molecules in postmenopausal women on hormone replacement therapy and at risk for coronary artery disease. *Metabolism.* 2004; 53:377-381.

[4]Oscai LB, Patterson JA, Bogard DL, Beck Rothermel BL. Normalization of serum triglycerides and lipoprotein electrophoretic patterns by exercise. *American Journal of Cardiology.* 1972; 30:775-780.

[5]Powers SK, Ji LL, Leeuwenburgh C. Exercise training-induced alterations in skeletal muscle antioxidant capacity: a brief review. *Medical and Science in Sports and Exercise.* 1999; 31:987-997.

[6]Smith JK, Dykes R, Douglas JE, Krishnaswamy G, Berk S. Long-term exercise and atherogenic activity of blood mononuclear cells in persons at risk of developing ischemic heart disease. *Journal of the American Medical Association.* 1999; 281:1722-1727.

[7]Hambrecht R, Work A, Gielen S, Linke A, et al. Effect of exercise on coronary endothelial function in patients with coronary artery disease. *New England Journal of Medicine.* 2000; 342:454-460.

[8]Hambrecht R, Walther C, Mobius-Winkler S, Linke A, et al. Percutaneous coronary angioplasty compared with exercise training in patients with stable coronary artery disease: a randomized trial. *Circulation.* 2004; 109:1371-1378.

[9]Powell KE, Thompson PD, Caspersen CJ, Kendrick JS. Physical activity and the incidence of coronary heart disease. *Annual Review of Public Health.* 1987; 8:253-287.

[10]Paffenbarger Jr RS, Hede RT, Wing AL, Hsieh CC. Physical activity, all-cause mortality and longevity of college alumni. *New England Journal of Medicine.* 1986; 314:605-613.

[11]Tanasescu M, Leitzmann MF, RimmEf, Willett WC, et al. Exercise type and intensity in relation to coronary heart disease in men. *Journal of the American Medical Association.* 2002; 288:1994-2000.

Chapter 9

[1]Ornish D, *Love and Survival.* (New York: HarperCollins, 1998).

[2]Egolf B, Lasker S, Wolf D, Potvin L. Featuring the health risks and mortality: The Roseto Effect. A 50-year comparison of mortality rates. *American Journal of Public Health.* 1992; 82(8): 1089-92.

[3]Wolf S. Predictors of myocardial infarction over a span of 30 years in Roseto, Pennsylvania. *Integrative Physiological & Behavioral Science.* 1992; 27(3): 246-57.

[4]Marmot MG, Syme SL, Kagan A. Epidemiologic studies of coronary heart disease and stroke in Japanese men living in Japan, Hawaii, and California: Prevalence of coronary and hypertensive heart disease and associated risk factors. *American Journal of Epidemiology.* 1975; 102(6): 514-25.

[5]Marmot MG, Syme SL. Acculturation and coronary heart disease in Japanese-Americans. *American Journal of Epidemiology.* 1976; 104(3): 225-47.

[6]Ruberman W, Weinblatt E, Goldberg D, and Chaudhary BS. Psychosocial influences on mortality after myocardial infarction. *New England Journal of Medicine.* 1984; 311(9): 552-59.

[7]Kaplan G, Salonen R, Cohen D. Social connections and mortality from all causes and from cardiovascular disease: Prospective evidence from Eastern Finland. *American Journal of Epidemiology.* 1988; 128(2): 370-80.

[8]Schoenbach VJ, Kaplan BH, Fredman L, Kleinbaum DG. Social ties and mortality in Evans County, Georgia. *American Journal of Epidemiology.* 1986; 123(4): 577-91.

[9]Oxman TE, Freeman DH, Manheimer ED. Lack of social participation or religious strength and comfort as risk factors for death after cardiac surgery in the elderly. *Psychosomatic Medicine.* 1995; 57:5-15.

[10]Seeman TE, Syme SL. Social networks and coronary artery disease: A comparison of the structure and function of social relations as predictors of disease. *Psychosomatic Medicine.* 1987; 49(4): 341-54.

[11]Horsten M, Kirkeeide R, Svane B, Schenck-Gustafsson, et al. Social support and coronary artery disease in women in *Love and Intimacy* by Dean Ornish (HarperCollins: New York, 1998).

[12]Williams RB, Barefoot R, Califf M. Prognostic importance of social and economic resources among medically treated patients with angiographically documented coronary artery disease. *Journal of the American Medical Association.* 1992; 267(4): 520-24.

[13]Medalie JH, Goldbourt U. Angina pectoris among 10,000 men. II. Psychosocial and other risk factors as evidenced by a multivariate analysis of a five year incidence study. *American Journal of Medicine.* 1976; 60(6): 910-21.

[14]Wiklund I, Oden A, Sanne H. Prognostic importance of somatic and psychosocial variables after a first myocardial infarction. *American Journal of Epidemiology.* 1982; 115(5): 684-94.

[15]Chandra V, Szklo M, Goldberg R. The impact of marital status on survival after an acute myocardial infarction: A population-based study. *American Journal of Epidemiology.* 1983; 117(3): 320-25.

[16]Case RB, Moss AJ, Case N. Living alone after myocardial infarction. Impact on prognosis. *Journal of the American Medical Association.* 1992; 267(4): 515-19.

[17]Berkman L, Leo-Summers L, Horwitz RI. Emotional support and survival after myocardial infarction. A prospective population-based study of the elderly. *Annals of Internal Medicine.* 1992; 117(12): 1003-9.

[18]Friedmann E, Thomas SA. Pet ownership, social support, and one-year survival after acute myocardial infarction in the Cardiac Arrhythmia Suppression Trial (CAST). *American Journal of Cardiology.* 1995; 76:1213-17.

[19]Friedmann E, Katcher A, Lynch J. Animal companions and one-year survival of patients after discharge from a coronary care unit. *Public Health Reports.* 1980; 95:307-12.

[20]Friedmann E, Katcher A, Thomas SA. Social interaction and blood pressure: Influence of animal companions. *Journal of Nervous and Mental Disease.* 1983; 171:461-65.

[21]Siegel JM. Stressful life events and use of physician services among the elderly: The moderating role of pet ownership. *Journal of Personality and Social Psychology.* 1990; 58:1081-86.

[22]Wassertheil-Smoller S, Shumaker S, Ockene J, et al. Depression and cardiovascular sequelae in postmenopausal women: The Women's Health Initiative (WHI). *Archives of Internal Medicine.* 2004; 164:289.

[23]Ariyo AA, Haan M, Tangen CM, et al. Depressive symptoms and risks of coronary heart disease and mortality in elderly Americans. *Circulation*. 2000; 102:1773.

[24]Pratt LA, Ford DE, Crum RM, et al. Depression, psychotropic medication, and risk of myocardial infarction. Prospective data from the Baltimore ECA follow-up. *Circulation*. 1996; 94:3123.

[25]Applegate WB, Pressel S, Wittes J, et al. Impact of the treatment of isolated systolic hypertension on behavioral variables: Results from the Systolic Hypertension in the Elderly Program (SHEP) Study. *Archives of Internal Medicine*. 1994; 154:2154.

[26]Penninx BWJH, Guralnik JM, Mendes de Leon CF, et al. Cardiovascular events and mortality and newly and chronically depressed persons >70 years of age. *American Journal of Cardiology*. 1998; 81:988.

[27]Parkes CM, Benjamin B, Fitzgerald RG. Broken heart: A statistical study of increased mortality among widowers. *British Medical Journal*. 1969; 1:740.

[28]Mittleman MA, Maclure M, Sherwood JB, et al. Death of a significant person increased the risk of acute MI onset (abstract). *Circulation*. 1996; 93:621A.

[29]Tofler GH, Stone PH, Maclure M, et al. Analysis of possible triggers of acute myocardial infarction (the MILIS Study). *American Journal of Cardiology*. 1990; 66:22.

[30]Myers R, Dewar HA. Circumstances surrounding sudden deaths from coronary artery disease with coroner's necropsies. *British Heart Journal*. 1975; 37:1133.

[31]Behar S, Halabi M, Reicher-Reiss H, et al. Circadian variation and possible external triggers of onset of myocardial infarction. *American Journal of Medicine*. 1993 Apr 9; 4(4):395-400.

[32]Shekelle RB, Gale M, Ostfeld AM, et al. Hostility, risk of coronary disease and mortality. *Psychosomatic Medicine*. 1983; 45:109.

[33]Miller TQ, Smith TW, Turner CW, et al. A meta-analytic review of research on hostility and physical health. *Psychological Bulletin*. 1996; 119:322-48.

[34]Mittleman MA, Maclure M, Sherwood JB, et al. Triggering of acute myocardial infarction onset by episodes of anger. Determinants of Myocardial Infarction Onset Investigators. *Circulation*. 1995; 92:1720.

[35]Kawachi I, Colditz GA, Ascherio A, et al. Prospective study of phobic anxiety and risk of coronary heart disease in men. Circulation. 1994; 89:1992.

Chapter 10

Newman TB, Hulley SB. Carcinogenicity of lipid-lowering drugs. *Journal of the American Medical Association.* 1993; 13:571-578.

[2]Ornish D, Scherwitz LW, Billings JH, et al. Intensive lifestyle changes for reversal of coronary heart disease. *Journal of the American Medical Association.* 1998 Dec 16; 280(23): 2001-2007.

[3]Barnard RJ, Guzy PM, Rosenberg JM, Trexler O'Brien L. Effects of an intensive exercise and nutrition program on patients with coronary artery disease: five-year follow up. *Journal of Cardiopulmonary Rehabilitation.* 1983; 3:183-190.

[4]Roberts CK, Barnard RJ. Effects of exercise and diet on chronic disease. *Journal of Applied Physiology.* 2005; 98:3-30.

INDEX

———

O

oil
    canola 159
    fish 158
    olive 158
    omega-6 158
    polyunsaturated 154
    saturated 156
    trans 154
oils
    partially hydrogenated 141
olive oil 158
Orme-Johnson, David 127
Ornish, Dean 208
oxy-cholesterol
    cell-damaging effects 140
    food sources 141
    heat, and 141

P

Pasteur 29
Paterson, J.C. 44
Pfrieger, B. 19
policolsanol 213
Posicor 112
potato chips 13
Pravachol 101
pravastatin 101
prc-diabetes 64
primary prevention trials 91
Pritikin, Nathan 209
Propulsid 112
protein theory 33

R

Ravnskov, Uffe 38
red rice yeast 213
relative risk 72
Rezulin 111
rhabdomyalosis 24
Rhinehard, James 145

T

Transcendental Meditation
    aging, and 131
    Canadian health care utilization, and 129
    heart disease reduction, and 128
    insurance cost reductions, and 127
    multimodal heart program, and 211
    National Institutes of Health (NIH) research on 130
    smoking, and 131
trans-oils 154, 155

V

vegetarian diet
    advantages of 149
    protein deficiency, and 149
Vioxx 110
Virchow, Rudolph 31, 64, 145
vitamin C 58
vitamin E 57
vitamins
    losses with over-processing 150

W

weight training 180
West of Scotland Coronary Prevention Study Group (WOSCOPS). See WOSCOPS Trial
WHO Cooperative Trial 91
WISE study 61
World Health Organization (WHO) Cooperative Trial. See WHO Cooperative Trial
WOSCOPS 164
WOSCOPS Trial 92, 94

Z

Zocor 20, 100, 206